VOLUME 2

RADIOGRAPHIC ANATOMY, POSITIONING, & PROCEDURES WORKBOOK

*This workbook is dedicated to the most important person in my life,
my wife, Sharon Hayes. Her love and support for me have created all the happiness
in my life. She was the motivation that inspired me to become
a radiologic technology educator, and she is the reason I still pursue goals;
therefore, this publication is for her.*

VOLUME 2

RADIOGRAPHIC ANATOMY, POSITIONING, & PROCEDURES WORKBOOK

Third Edition

Steven G. Hayes, Sr., BSRT, MEd, RT(R)

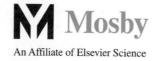

Mosby

An Affiliate of Elsevier Science

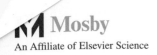

An Affiliate of Elsevier Science

11830 Westline Industrial Drive
St. Louis, Missouri 63146

NOTICE

Radiography is an ever-changing field. Standard safety precautions must be followed, but as new research and clinical experience broaden our knowledge, changes in treatment and drug therapy may become necessary or appropriate. Readers are advised to check the most current product information provided by the manufacturer of each drug to be administered to verify the recommended dose, the method and duration of administration, and contraindications. It is the responsibility of the licensed prescriber, relying on experience and knowledge of the patient, to determine dosages and the best treatment for each individual patient. Neither the publisher nor the author assumes any liability for any injury and/or damage to persons or property arising from this publication.

Previous editions copyrighted 1996, 1999

International Standard Book Number 0-323-01481-X

Acquisitions Editor: Jeanne Wilke
Editorial Assistant: Paige Mosher
Project Manager: Joy Moore
Senior Designer: Mark A. Oberkrom

Printed in the United States of America

Last digit is the print number: 9   8   7   6   5   4   3   2   1

Preface

This two-volume workbook has been developed to accompany *Mosby's Radiographic Instructional Series (MRIS): Anatomy, Positioning, and Procedures* multimedia and *Merrill's Atlas of Radiographic Positions and Radiologic Procedures* (commonly referred to as *Merrill's Atlas* or just, *Merrill's*). The chapters in this workbook are presented in the same order as the 27 units in *Mosby's Radiographic Instructional Series: Anatomy, Positioning, and Procedures* multimedia and the first 27 chapters of *Merrill's Atlas of Radiographic Positions and Radiologic Procedures*. However, the material presented in this workbook can function as a useful review for any anatomy and positioning course or as a review for the certification exam. The exercises found in this workbook are designed to give you a thorough review of osteology, anatomy, physiology, arthrology, and radiographic examinations.

The following features were revised or newly added to the second edition.

• Updated and standardized anatomy terminology to reflect the usage in *Merrill's Atlas* as well as the most current anatomy texts and *Nomina Anatomica*
• New questions on computed radiography (CR), including the slight positioning changes and the kVp setting changes necessary for CR
• New exercise sections on radiographic quality in Chapter 1, identifying projections of the vertebral column in Chapter 8, and review of essential mammographic projections in Chapter 24
• New chapter review self-tests for Chapters 20 through 23
• More film evaluations, offering additional opportunities to evaluate images for proper positioning
• More positioning questions to complement the workbook's strong anatomy review
• Reformatted exercises for ease of writing in answers while working through the MRIS multimedia tutorials

The following features have been revised or newly added to the third edition.

• More than 60 new pictures, radiographic images, and illustrations
• New matching exercises for pathology terms in 12 chapters that have essential projections
• New exercises for identifying projections of the upper limb in Chapter 4, for identifying projections of the shoulder girdle in Chapter 5, and for identifying mammographic projections in Chapter 24
• New review exercises for the tangential projection for the intertubercular groove in Chapter 5 and for the verticosubmental projection for the cranium in Chapter 20

• New review exercises for the completely revised Chapter 13, "Trauma Radiography"
• Improved sequencing of exercise items with the text of *Merrill's Atlas of Radiographic Positions and Radiologic Procedures*
• Numerous exercises updated to reflect related changes found in the current edition of *Merrill's Atlas of Radiographic Positions and Radiologic Procedures*
• Chapter 24, Mammography, expanded to seven separate exercises from its original three exercises

All chapters that have essential projections are divided into two sections: (1) an anatomy section and (2) a positioning section.

• The anatomy sections consist of various exercises such as labeling and identification diagrams, short-answer and multiple-choice questions, matching exercises, and crossword puzzles.
• The positioning sections include short-answer and multiple-choice questions, true-false statements, fill-in-the-blank statements, matching exercises, identification exercises, and radiographic comparisons of standard radiographic projections.
• At the end of each chapter is a collection of multiple-choice questions that reviews the entire chapter.
• Answers for all exercises are provided at the end of each volume.

Some of the radiographic projections included and described in *Merrill's Atlas* are for reference purposes only and are no longer routinely performed in radiologic imaging facilities. Therefore, we have chosen to focus on essential terminology, anatomy, and positioning information for the projections identified as necessary for entry-level competency as determined by a survey of radiologic technology programs in the United States and Canada. For more information on the survey consult the Preface contained in *Merrill's Atlas*.

Some chapters of *Merrill's Atlas* (Volumes 1 and 2) have limited radiographic applications or consist of radiographic procedures only rarely performed today because of technological advances in adjunct medical imagery modalities (e.g., computed tomography, magnetic resonance imaging, and diagnostic ultrasound). Because those chapters do not include radiographic examinations deemed essential for entry-level competency, this workbook provides only cursory coverage for those chapters.

To use this workbook most effectively you should first study the appropriate anatomic and radiographic sections from *Merrill's Atlas* and the multimedia series. Then complete the exercises that relate to the chapter of interest.

Steven G. Hayes, Sr.

Acknowledgments

My appreciation is extended to those who were instrumental in the development of this workbook. The first, of course, is my wife Sharon. The simple dedication in the front of this workbook does not adequately express my appreciation for all her support and assistance with this publication and with every goal I have ever pursued. For more than 30 years, she has given me more than I can ever return in kind.

The difficulties of a major writing project are, sometimes, not fully realized by an author on initially accepting the task. Support from family members can often affect how successful an author is in completing a publication. I am fortunate to have the complete support of my family. For that reason, I need to recognize my two children, who allowed me to temporarily withdraw my presence from their activities. My son, Steven G. Hayes, Jr., ASRT, RT(R) (ARRT), is very supportive of everything I do, especially with the development of this workbook. Because he is an experienced radiologic educator and technologist, his knowledge of radiographic positioning was very beneficial to me in obtaining some of the radiographic images I needed and with assisting in the development of the text. I value his support and advice. I also want to thank my daughter, Tonya, for her understanding when I was excusing myself from family activities so I could sustain my production schedule. To both, I apologize for depriving them of my time during the development of this workbook.

Another radiologic educator, Jackie Miller, BSRT, RT(R) (ARRT), has been a close friend and colleague of mine longer than either of us can remember. I know no one who has more common sense than Jackie. Other than my wife, he probably knows me better than does anyone else. I appreciate his assistance with obtaining some of the radiographs used in this workbook and the long-term encouragement he has given me in all my endeavors.

I also want to recognize my Mosby editors, Jeanne Wilke, Lisa Potts, and Carole Glauser. Jeanne is the acquisitions editor who first proposed this workbook project to me. I appreciate the confidence she had in me from the very onset. Lisa, an accomplished developmental editor, was very important in assisting me throughout the entire development of the first edition of this workbook. She was always available to answer every question I had and provided useful advice that made my work so much easier. Thank you, Lisa. For the preparation of the second edition, I thank Carole Glauser for coordinating the many activities that transform a manuscript into the finished publication.

I also thank Philip W. Ballinger, MS, RT, FAERS, and Eugene Frank, MA, RT(R), FASRT, co-authors for *Merrill's Atlas of Radiographic Positions and Radiologic Procedures,* ninth edition. Philip was quick to answer my technical questions concerning *Merrill's Atlas* and offered significant suggestions. For the preparation of the second edition, in addition to Philip, I thank Eugene for his replies to the countless e-mail messages I sent him almost nightly for months as the revision neared its completion.

For the preparation of the second edition, in addition to the preceding, I sincerely appreciate the comments and suggestions from students, educators, and reviewers. Their collective input helped make this workbook a better learning aid.

For the preparation of the third edition I want to specifically thank Eugene Frank, MA, RT(R), FASRT, author of *Merrill's Atlas of Radiographic Positions and Radiologic Procedures,* tenth edition. In addition to some face-to-face meetings, almost daily we sent e-mail messages between us to ensure that our publications are the highest quality possible and that essential information is identical in both our publications. He is a constant source of technical expertise for me, and his suggestions immensely helped me throughout the writing of this edition. Additionally, my sincere appreciation is extended to Jeanne Wilke, Executive Editor, for her continual support and management strategies in all aspects of the production of this workbook. One valuable service Jeanne provided me was ensuring that I always had very competent editorial assistants and developmental editors throughout the development of this edition. Specifically, Jennifer Genett and Rebecca Swisher, Developmental Editors, and Melissa Kuster and Paige Mosher, Editorial Assistants, provided important services during this revision project. Jennifer was in on the initial planning stages, Melissa helped with the illustrations and figures, and Paige and Rebecca coordinated all the end activities that culminate with the final printed product. To those four ladies I offer my sincere appreciation for their constant efforts to keep this edition moving along by taking care of so many tasks that authors are unable to do for themselves.

I have been lucky to have the love and support of many wonderful people. Those I have just mentioned are the ones who really are responsible for this workbook.

Steven G. Hayes, Sr.

Contents

CHAPTER 14

Mouth and Salivary Glands

Review

Instructions: This exercise provides an anatomic review of the mouth and salivary glands and a cursory review of sialography. Identify structures, fill in missing words, provide a short answer, match columns, select the best choice, or choose true or false (explaining any statement you believe to be false) for each item.

1. Identify each lettered structure shown in Fig. 14-1.

   A. _____

   B. _____

   C. _____

   D. _____

   E. _____

   F. _____

   G. _____

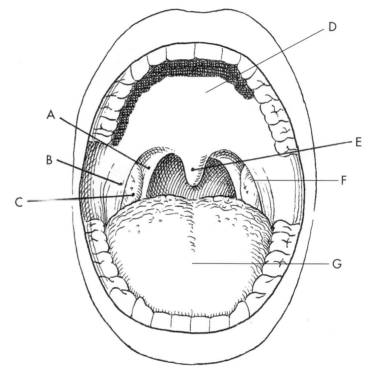

Figure 14-1 Anterior aspect of the oral cavity.

2. Identify each lettered structure shown in Fig. 14-2.

A. _____

B. _____

C. _____

D. _____

3. Identify each lettered structure shown in Fig. 14-3.

A. _____

B. _____

C. _____

D. _____

E. _____

F. _____

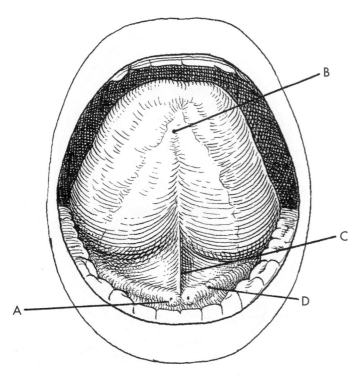

Figure 14-2 Anterior view of the undersurface of tongue and floor of mouth.

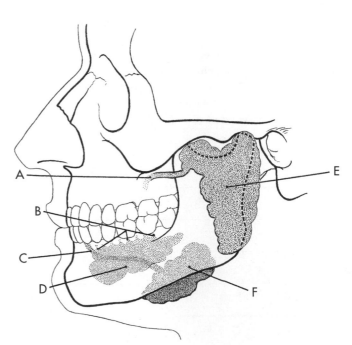

Figure 14-3 The salivary glands from the left lateral aspect.

4. Identify each lettered structure shown in Fig. 14-4.

A. _____

B. _____

C. _____

D. _____

E. _____

F. _____

G. _____

5. Identify each lettered structure shown in Fig. 14-5.

A. _____

B. _____

C. _____

D. _____

E. _____

F. _____

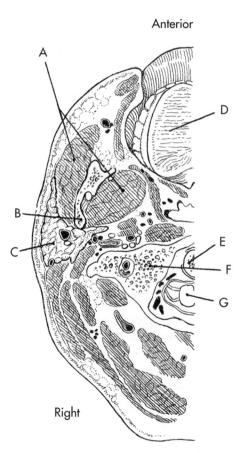

Figure 14-4 Horizontal section of the face showing the relation of the parotid gland to the mandibular ramus.

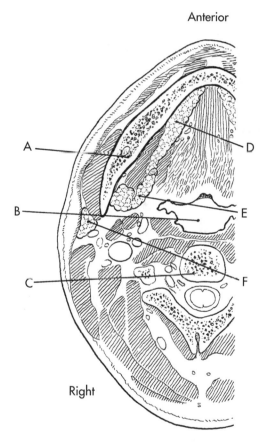

Figure 14-5 Horizontal section of the face showing the relation of the submandibular and sublingual glands to surrounding structures.

6. What is the first division of the digestive system?

   _____

7. Define mastication.

8. Which structures function in mastication?

   _____

9. What is the purpose of saliva?

10. Name the three pairs of salivary glands.

11. Define sialography.

12. What type of contrast medium is used for sialography?

   _____

13. Why can only one salivary gland at a time be examined by the sialographic method?

14. List two reasons why preliminary radiographs are made before the introduction of the contrast medium.

15. Name the three projections that demonstrate the salivary glands and ducts.

16. Which salivary glands are demonstrated with the axial projection (intraoral method)?
    a. Parotid and sublingual
    b. Parotid and submandibular
    c. Sublingual and submandibular

17. Which sialographic projection is the only projection that demonstrates an unobstructed image of the sublingual gland area?
    a. Lateral
    b. Tangential
    c. Axial (intraoral method)

18. Which sialographic image can be made with occlusal film?
    a. Lateral
    b. Tangential
    c. Axial (intraoral method)

19. Which sialographic projection directs the central ray along the lateral surface of the mandibular ramus?
    a. Lateral
    b. Tangential
    c. Axial (intraoral method)

20. True or False. The patient may be positioned prone or supine for the tangential projection.

21. True or False. The mandibular ramus should be parallel with the plane of the image receptor (IR) for the tangential projection.

22. True or False. Parotid glands on both sides of the face should be demonstrated with the same tangential exposure.

23. Examine Fig. 14-6 and answer the questions that follow.

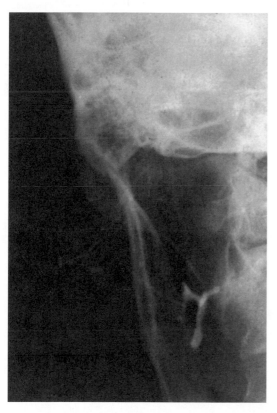

Figure 14-6 Sialogram showing opacification of a gland.

a. Which projection does this image represent?

_____

b. Which salivary gland is demonstrated?

_____

c. What is the special breathing technique that can be performed by the patient to improve the radiographic demonstration of the gland with this type of projection?

_____

24. Examine Fig. 14-7 and answer the questions that follow.

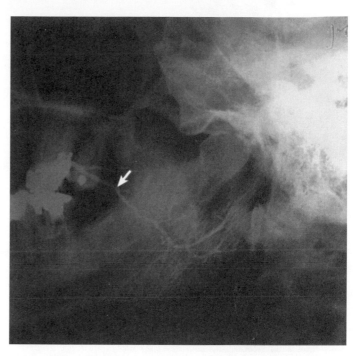

Figure 14-7 Sialogram showing opacification of a gland.

a. Which projection does this image represent?

_____

b. Which salivary gland is demonstrated?

_____

c. To which duct does the arrow point?

_____

25. Examine Fig. 14-8 and answer the questions that follow.

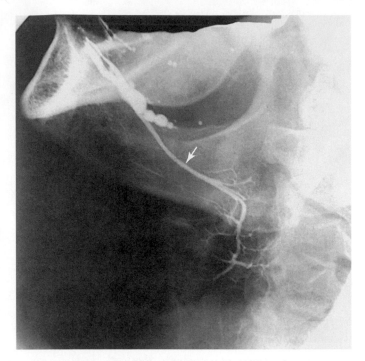

Figure 14-8 Sialogram showing opacification of a gland.

a. Which projection does this image represent?

_____

b. Which salivary gland is demonstrated?

_____

c. To which duct does the arrow point?

_____

Self-Test: Mouth and Salivary Glands

Instructions: Answer the following questions by selecting the best choice.

1. What is the first division of the digestive system?

   a. Mouth
   b. Stomach
   c. Small intestine
   d. Salivary glands

2. Which salivary gland is the largest?

   a. Parotid
   b. Sublingual
   c. Submandibular

3. Which salivary glands are the smallest?

   a. Parotid
   b. Sublingual
   c. Submandibular

4. Which salivary glands are located along the lateral aspect of the mandibular ramus?

   a. Parotid
   b. Sublingual
   c. Submandibular

5. Which two imaging modalities have greatly reduced the frequency of sialography?

   a. Computed tomography and ultrasonography
   b. Computed tomography and magnetic resonance imaging
   c. Conventional tomography and ultrasonography
   d. Conventional tomography and magnetic resonance imaging

6. For sialography, into which structure is the contrast medium injected?

   a. Vein
   b. Artery
   c. Muscle
   d. Salivary duct

7. Which sialographic projection directs the central ray along the mandibular ramus?

   a. Lateral projection
   b. Tangential projection
   c. Verticosubmental projection
   d. Axial projection (intraoral method)

8. Which sialographic projection demonstrates a parotid gland superimposed over a mandibular ramus?

   a. Lateral projection
   b. Tangential projection
   c. Verticosubmental projection
   d. Axial projection (intraoral method)

9. Which two sialographic projections best demonstrate the parotid gland?

   a. Axial and lateral projections
   b. Axial and verticosubmental projections
   c. Tangential and lateral projections
   d. Tangential and verticosubmental projections

10. Which sialographic projection demonstrates an unobstructed view of the sublingual area?

    a. Lateral projection
    b. Tangential projection
    c. Verticosubmental projection
    d. Axial projection (intraoral method)

11. Which gland is demonstrated with tangential projections?

    a. Parotid
    b. Sublingual
    c. Submandibular

12. Which sialographic projection demonstrates parotid and submandibular glands?

    a. Lateral projection
    b. Tangential projection
    c. Axial projection (intraoral method)

13. Which salivary gland can be demonstrated with a lateral projection when the patient's head is adjusted so that the midsagittal plane is rotated approximately 15 degrees toward the IR from true lateral and the central ray is directed to a point 1 inch (2.5 cm) above the mandibular ramus?

    a. Parotid
    b. Sublingual
    c. Submandibular

14. Which salivary gland can be demonstrated with a lateral projection when the patient's head is positioned true lateral and a perpendicular central ray is directed to the inferior margin of the mandibular angle?

    a. Parotid
    b. Sublingual
    c. Submandibular

15. For the lateral projection demonstrating the submandibular gland, what is the purpose of pressing the tongue to the floor of the mouth?

    a. To hold the intraoral film in place
    b. To displace the submandibular gland below the mandible
    c. To prevent the tongue from superimposing the submandibular gland

CHAPTER 15

Anterior Part of the Neck

Review

Instructions: This exercise is a review of the anatomy and radiography of the anterior part of the neck. Identify structures, fill in missing words, or provide a short answer for each item.

1. Identify each lettered structure shown in Fig. 15-1.

   A. _____ Nasal septum _____

   B. _____ Nasopharynx _____

   C. _____ Uvula _____

   D. _____ Epiglottis _____

   E. _____ Vocal folds _____

   F. _____ Larynx _____

   G. _____ Laryngeal pharynx _____

   H. _____ Soft palate _____

   I. _____ Piriform Recess _____

   J. _____ Rima glottidis _____

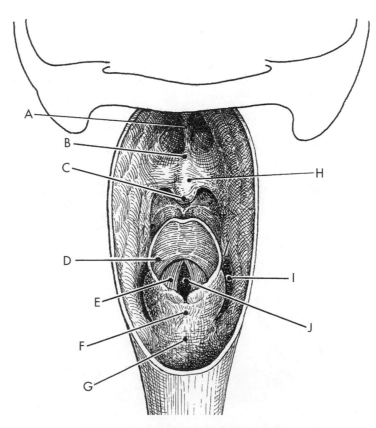

Figure 15-1 posterior view of the neck.

2. Identify each lettered structure shown in Fig. 15-2.

A. _____ Soft palate _____

B. _____ Nasopharynx _____

C. _____ Uvula _____

D. _____ Oropharynx _____

E. _____ Epiglottis _____

F. _____ Vocal cords _____

G. _____ Larynx _____

H. _____ Hard palate _____

I. _____ Hyoid bone _____

J. _____ Laryngeal pharynx _____

K. _____ Trachea _____

L. _____ Thyroid Cartilage _____

M. _____ Esophagus _____

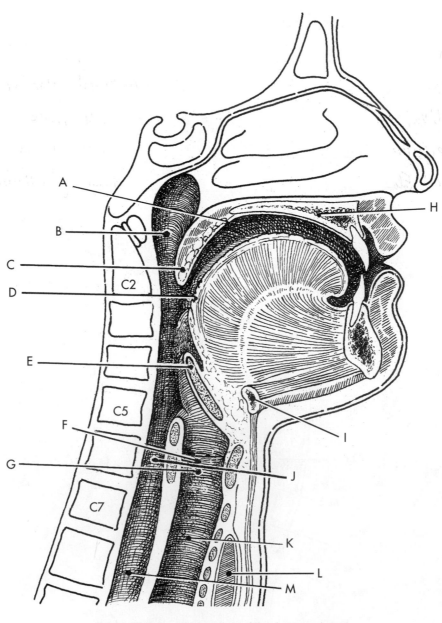

Figure 15-2 Sagittal section of the face and neck.

3. Identify each lettered structure shown in Fig. 15-3.

A. _____Superior Parathyroid gland_____

B. _____Thyroid gland_____

C. _____INF. Parathyroid gland_____

D. _____Esophagus_____

E. _____Thyroid Cartilage_____

F. _____Isthmus of thyroid_____

G. _____Trachea_____

4. Identify each lettered structure shown in Fig. 15-4.

A. _____Hyoid Bone_____

B. _____Thyroid Cartilage_____

C. _____Trachea_____

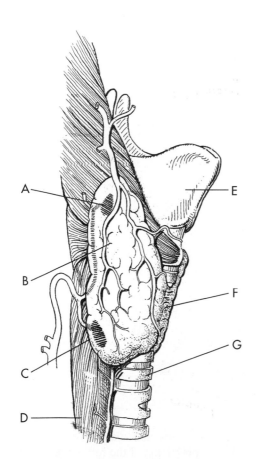

Figure 15-3 Lateral aspect of the laryngeal area.

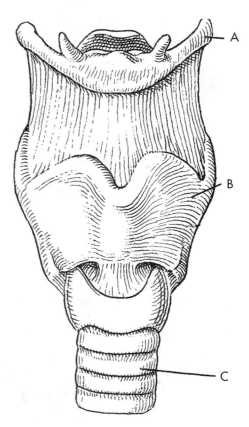

Figure 15-4 Anterior aspect of the larynx.

5. Identify each lettered structure shown in Fig. 15-5.

A. _____ Base of Tongue _____

B. _____ Epiglottis _____

C. _____ Vestibular Fold (false Vocal Cord) _____

D. _____ Rima glottidis (open) _____

E. _____ Rima glottidis (closed) _____

F. _____ Vocal fold (true vocal cord) _____

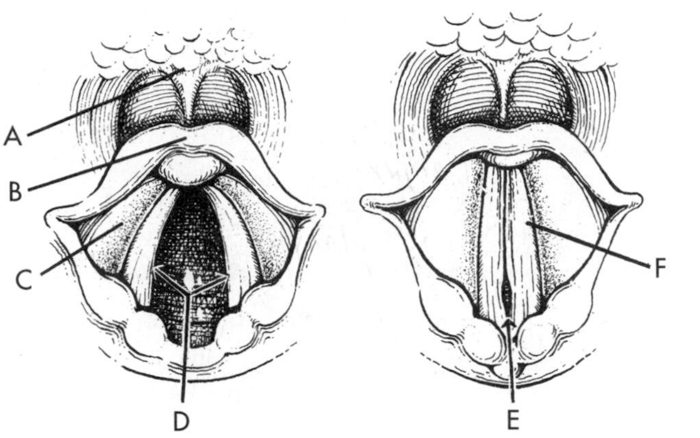

Figure 15-5 Superior aspect of the larynx (open and closed true vocal folds).

6. For radiographic purposes, the neck is divided into _____ Post. _____ and _____ Ant _____ portions.

7. The upper part of the respiratory system located in the anterior part of the neck is the _____ trachea _____.

8. The upper part of the digestive system located in the anterior part of the neck is the _____ Esophagus _____.

9. The two major glands located in the anterior part of the neck are the _____ thyroid _____ gland and the _____ parathyroid _____ gland.

10. The structure of the upper neck that serves as a passage for both food and air and is common to the respiratory and digestive systems is the _____ pharynx _____.

11. The portion of the pharynx located above the soft palate is the _____ Nasopharynx _____

12. The portion of the pharynx located from the soft palate to the hyoid bone is the _____ Oropharynx _____.

13. The organ of voice is the _____ Larynx _____.

14. The structure that comprises the vocal apparatus of the larynx is the _____ glottis _____.

15. The projections that demonstrate the pharynx and larynx are _____ AP _____ and _____ LAT. _____.

16. During what four bodily functions are radiographs of the pharynx and larynx made?

_____ Breathing, phonation, stress maneuvers, swallowing _____

17. Identify the body position in which the patient should be placed for each of the following examinations of the pharynx and larynx:

a. Tomographic studies: _____ Supine _____

b. AP and lateral projections: _____ upright _____

18. For the AP projection, the central ray should be directed perpendicular to the _____ Laryngeal _____ _____ prominence _____.

19. Identify the x-ray tube and image receptor centering points for the lateral projection of the following structures:

a. Nasopharynx: _____ Level of EAM _____

b. Oropharynx: _____ Level of mandibular Angles _____

c. Larynx: _____ Level of the Laryngeal prominence _____

20. Identify each lettered structure shown in Fig. 15-6.

A. _____ Air - filled pharynx _____

B. _____ Hyoid _____

C. _____ Laryngeal structures _____

D. _____ trachea _____

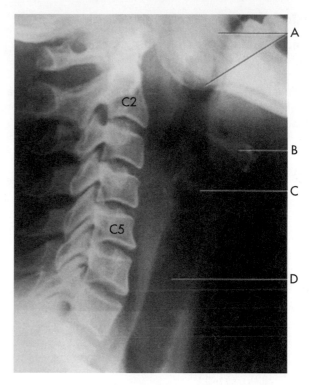

Figure 15-6 Lateral pharynx and larynx (Valsalva maneuver).

Self-Test: Anterior Part of the Neck

Instructions: Answer the following questions by selecting the best choice.

1. What is the musculomembranous tubular structure located in front of the vertebrae and behind the nose, the mouth, and the larynx?

   a. Glottis
   b. Trachea
   c. Pharynx
   d. Esophagus

2. Which structure of the neck is approximately 1½ inches (4 cm) in length and is situated below the root of the tongue and in front of the laryngeal pharynx?

   a. Larynx
   b. Trachea
   c. Esophagus
   d. Oropharynx

3. Which structure forms the laryngeal prominence?

   a. Epiglottis
   b. True vocal cord
   c. Cricoid cartilage
   d. Thyroid cartilage

4. Which structure prevents leakage into the larynx during swallowing?

   a. Pharynx
   b. Epiglottis
   c. Cricoid cartilage
   d. Thyroid cartilage

5. What is the most superiorly located structure of the neck?

   a. Larynx
   b. Glottis
   c. Pharynx
   d. Epiglottis

6. For the AP projection that demonstrates the pharynx and larynx, to which level of the patient should the central ray be directed?

   a. C1
   b. C7
   c. Mandibular angles
   d. Laryngeal prominence

7. For preliminary AP and lateral projections that demonstrate the pharynx and larynx, when should the exposures be made to ensure filling the throat passages with air?

   a. During expiration
   b. During inspiration
   c. After suspended expiration
   d. After suspended inspiration

8. Which body position should be used for tomographic examinations of the pharynx and larynx?

   a. Prone
   b. Supine
   c. Upright lateral
   d. Recumbent lateral

9. For the lateral projection that demonstrates the oropharynx, to which level of the patient should the central ray be directed?

   a. C7
   b. Mandibular angles
   c. Laryngeal prominence
   d. External acoustic meatuses

10. Which procedure should the patient perform for tomographic studies of pharyngolaryngeal structures?

    a. Quiet inspiration through the nose
    b. Phonation of a high-pitched "e-e-e"
    c. Suspended respiration after expiration
    d. Suspended respiration after inspiration

CHAPTER 16

Digestive System: Abdomen, Liver, Spleen, and Biliary Tract

SECTION 1

Anatomy of the Abdomen, Liver, Spleen, and Biliary Tract

Exercise 1

Instructions: This exercise pertains to the abdominal contents. Identify structures for each question.

1. Identify each lettered structure shown in Fig. 16-1.

A. _____

B. _____

C. _____

D. _____

E. _____

F. _____

G. _____

H. _____

I. _____

J. _____

K. _____

L. _____

M. _____

N. _____

O. _____

P. _____

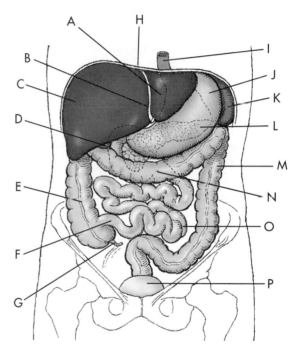

Figure 16-1 Anterior aspect of the abdominal viscera.

2. Identify each lettered structure shown in Fig. 16-2.

A. _____

B. _____

C. _____

D. _____

E. _____

F. _____

G. _____

H. _____

I. _____

J. _____

K. _____

L. _____

M. _____

N. _____

O. _____

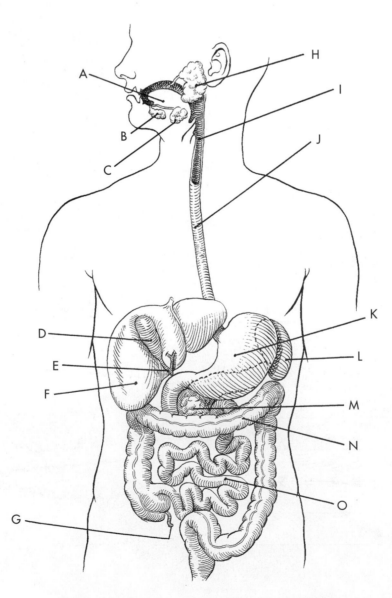

Figure 16-2 Alimentary tract and its accessory organs.

3. Identify each lettered structure shown in Fig. 16-3.

A. _____   I. _____

B. _____   J. _____

C. _____   K. _____

D. _____   L. _____

E. _____   M. _____

F. _____   N. _____

G. _____   O. _____

H. _____

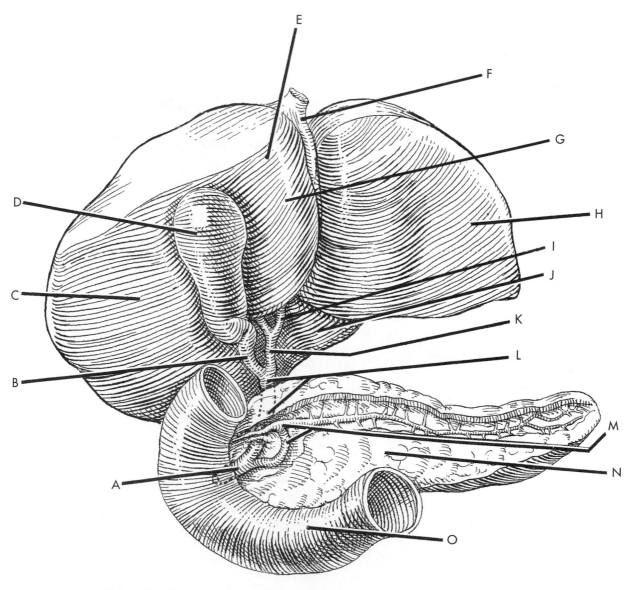

Figure 16-3 Visceral surface (inferoposterior aspect) of the liver and gallbladder.

4. Identify each lettered structure shown in Fig. 16-4.

A. _____

B. _____

C. _____

D. _____

E. _____

F. _____

G. _____

H. _____

I. _____

J. _____

5. Identify each lettered structure shown in Fig. 16-5.

A. _____

B. _____

C. _____

D. _____

E. _____

F. _____

G. _____

H. _____

I. _____

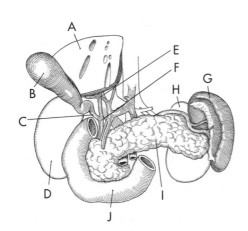

Figure 16-4 Visceral (inferoposterior) surface of gallbladder and bile ducts.

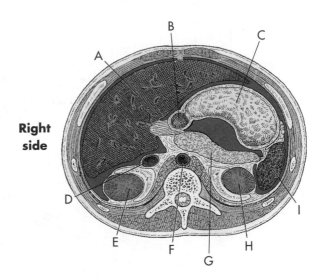

Figure 16-5 Sectional image of the upper abdomen showing the relationship of digestive system components.

Exercise 2

Match the pathology terms in Column A with the appropriate definition in Column B. Not all choices from Column B should be selected.

Column A

_____ 1. Ileus

_____ 2. Appendicitis

_____ 3. Cholecystitis

_____ 4. Cholelithiasis

_____ 5. Biliary stenosis

_____ 6. Ulcerative colitis

_____ 7 Bowel obstruction

_____ 8. Choledocholithiasis

_____ 9. Pneumoperitoneum

_____ 10. Abdominal aortic aneurysm

Column B

a. The presence of gallstones

b. Failure of bowel peristalsis

c. Narrowing of the bile ducts

d. Blockage of the bowel lumen

e. Inflammation of the appendix

f. Calculus in the common bile duct

g. Presence of air in the peritoneal cavity

h. Localized dilatation of the abdominal aorta

i. Acute or chronic inflammation of the gallbladder

j. Transfer of a cancerous lesion from one area to another

k. Recurrent disorder causing inflammatory ulceration in the colon

Exercise 3

Instructions: This exercise pertains to the liver, biliary system, pancreas, and spleen. Fill in missing words, provide a short answer, or choose true or false (explaining any statement you believe to be false) for each item.

1. The name of the double-walled seromembranous sac that lines the abdominal cavity is the _____.

2. The names of the two layers of the peritoneum are the _____ layer and the _____ layer.

3. The outer layer of the peritoneum that contacts the underside of the diaphragm is called the _____ layer.

4. The inner layer of the peritoneum that contacts various organs is called the _____ layer.

5. The organ that occupies most of the right hypochondrium and the epigastrium regions of the abdomen is the _____.

6. The largest organ in the abdominal cavity is the _____.

7. The radiographically significant physiologic function of the liver is the production of _____.

8. The right and left hepatic ducts join to form the _____ _____ _____.

9. The cystic duct enables bile from the liver to be stored in the _____.

10. The gallbladder is usually located on the inferior side of the right lobe of the _____.

11. The common hepatic duct unites with the cystic duct to form the _____ _____ _____.

12. In 20% of subjects, before entering the duodenum, the common bile duct joins with the _____ _____.

13. The muscular contraction of the gallbladder is activated by a hormone called _____.

14. Another name for the ampulla of Vater is the _____ _____.

15. The gland that produces insulin is the _____.

16. True or False. In a hypersthenic patient, the gallbladder is situated high and well away from the midsagittal plane.

17. True or False. The gallbladder is located posterior to the liver in the retroperitoneal space.

18. True or False. The pancreas cannot be demonstrated using plain radiography.

19. True or False. The spleen is an organ of the lymphatic system.

20. True or False. The pancreas and the liver secrete specialized digestive juices into the small intestine.

SECTION 2

Positioning of the Abdomen and Gallbladder

Exercise 1: Positioning for the Abdomen

Instructions: A variety of radiographic procedures are used to demonstrate the abdomen and its contents. A patient is usually first examined with plain radiography before specialized studies using contrast media are performed. This exercise reviews the positions and projections commonly used to produce radiographs of the abdomen without the introduction of a contrast medium. Fill in missing words, provide a short answer, select answers from a list, or choose true or false (explaining any statement you believe to be false) for each item.

Items 1 through 5 pertain to general procedures for abdominal radiography.

1. What three projections usually comprise the three-way or acute abdomen series?

    - *supine* KUB
    - AP ↑ ABD
    - PA chest

2. Why is a chest radiograph included as part of the acute abdomen series?

    - To demonstrate any free air that may be beneath the diaphragm

3. In the acute abdomen series, what radiograph should be substituted for the upright abdomen radiograph when the patient is unable to stand?

    - Lt. LAT. Decub.

4. List the three considerations for the use of gonadal shielding in abdominal radiography.

    - if gonads lie in close proximity (2") to primary x-ray field
    - if clinical objectives will not be compromised
    - if pt. has a reasonable reproductive potential

5. Visualizing the sharply defined outline of what muscle group is an excellent criterion for judging the quality of an abdomen radiograph?

    - Psoas major

Items 6 through 15 pertain to *anteroposterior* (AP) and *posteroanterior* (PA) projections. Examine Fig. 16-6 as you answer the following items.

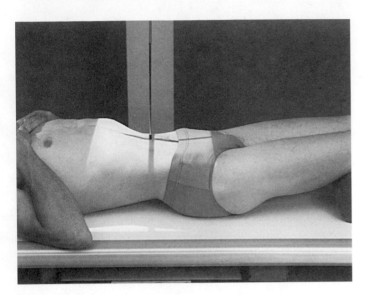

Figure 16-6 AP abdomen, supine.

6. What is the commonly used acronym that refers to the AP projection of the abdomen with the patient supine?

   KUB

7. Which plane of the body should be centered to the midline of the image receptor?

   Mid sagittal

8. For the AP projection with the patient supine, to what level of the patient should the image receptor (IR) be centered?

   iliac crest

9. List the two levels of the patient to which the IR should be centered when the patient is positioned upright, and give the reason for the difference in IR placement.

   - 2" ↑ crests - to include diaphragm
   - level of crest - to include bladder

10. What structure of the upper abdomen should be seen on the abdomen radiograph when the patient is upright? Explain why.

    - Diaphragm - to see if there is any free air beneath the diaphragm.

11. What breathing instructions should be given the patient?

    - Suspend respiration at the end of expiration

12. What is the advantage of exposing abdominal radiographs at the suspension of the recommended phase of respiration as compared to the other respiration phase?

    - so that abdominal organs are not compressed

13. What two identification markers should be seen on the radiograph when the patient is upright?

    - R or L marker
    - marker indicating the pt was upright

14. With reference to radiation protection, what is the advantage of the PA projection over the AP projection?

A Reduction in the radiation exp. to the gonads

15. From the following list, circle the three evaluation criteria that indicate the patient was properly positioned without rotation for a KUB radiograph.
    a. Intervertebral foramina should be open.
    b. Alae or wings of the ilia should be symmetric.
    c. Lumbar vertebrae pedicles should be superimposed.
    d. If seen, ischial spines of the pelvis should be symmetric.
    e. Spinous processes should be in the center of the lumbar vertebrae.

Items 16 through 26 pertain to the *AP projection, left lateral decubitus position.* Examine Fig. 16-7 as you answer the following items.

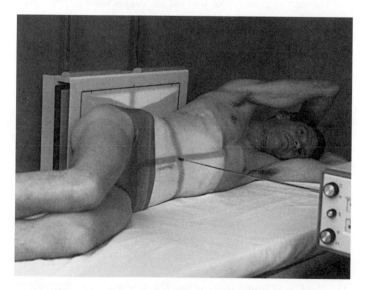

Figure 16-7 AP abdomen, left lateral decubitus position.

16. What is the advantage of the left lateral decubitus position compared to the supine position AP abdomen?

To Demonstrate Air - Fluid levels

17. Why is the left lateral decubitus position preferred over the right lateral decubitus position when the patient is unable to stand?

- To see Any free Air through the homogeneous background of the liver instead of being superimposed o air in stomach.

18. Describe the position of the patient for left lateral decubitus position.

- Pt recumbent in A Lat position - Lt. side ↓
- both Arms ↑, Knees Flexed

19. Why is it advisable to let the patient remain in the lateral recumbent position for several minutes before making the exposure?

- To Allow time for Any free air to rise to highest level in ABD.

20. With reference to the patient, describe the placement and centering of the image receptor.

- A vertically placed cassette should be centered Against the pt's post. side of ABD at the level of the iliac crests.

21. What breathing instructions should be given to the patient?

Suspend After expiration.

22. Describe how and to where the central ray should be directed.

⊥ to midpt. of cassette, entering at the level of the iliac crests.

23. Which side of the abdomen—the "up" side or the "down" side—should be demonstrated if only one side can be imaged and the patient is suspected of having fluid levels within the abdominal cavity?

Side ↓

24. Which side of the abdomen—the "up" side or the "down" side—should be demonstrated if only one side can be imaged and the patient may have free air in the abdomen?

Side ↑

25. What structure of the upper abdomen should be demonstrated on the radiograph?

Diaphragm

26. What identification markers should be seen on the radiograph?

—Markers indicating which side is ↑

Items 27 through 33 pertain to the *lateral projection*. Examine Fig. 16-8 as you answer the following items.

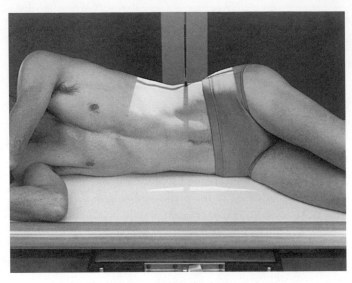

Figure 16-8 Right lateral abdomen.

27. (True) or False. A lateral projection of the abdomen can be performed with the patient placed in either the right lateral recumbent position or the left lateral recumbent position.

28. True or (False). The midsagittal plane should be perpendicular and centered to the IR.

29. True or (False). The exposure should be made after the patient has suspended respiration after full inspiration.

30. To what level of the patient should the IR be centered?

the iliac crests, or 2" ↑ iliac crest to include diaphragm

31. If a compression band is needed to immobilize the patient, where should it be placed?

Across the pelvis

32. Where exactly should the central ray enter the patient?

To A point on the midcoronal plane at the level of the iliac crests

33. What two areas of the image can be closely examined to determine if the patient was rotated?

Pelvis & lumbar vertebrae

Items 34 through 40 pertain to the *lateral projection, dorsal decubitus position*. Examine Fig. 16-9 as you answer the following items.

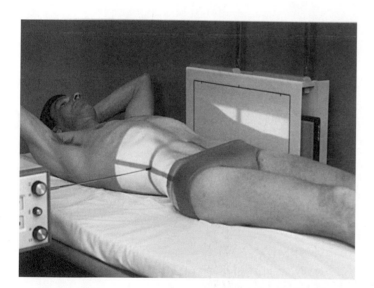

Figure 16-9 Lateral abdomen, left dorsal decubitus position.

34. What is the name of the radiographic position that produces a lateral image of the abdomen with the patient in the supine position?

Dorsal Decub.

35. What purpose is served by having the patient slightly flex his or her knees?

- To relieve strain on the pt.'s back by ↓ the lordotic curvature.

36. To what level of the patient should the long axis of the IR be centered?

Midcoronal plane.

37. How far above the level of the iliac crests should the central ray enter the patient?

2"

38. True or (False). The exposure should be made after the patient has suspended respiration at the end of inspiration.

39. (True) or False. The central ray should be directed horizontally and perpendicular relative to the center of the film.

40. From the following list, circle the three evaluation criteria that indicate the patient was correctly positioned for a lateral projection while placed in the dorsal decubitus position.

   a. The wings of the ilia should be symmetric.
   b. The entire abdomen should be demonstrated.
   c. The diaphragm should be included without motion.
   d. The abdominal contents should be seen with soft-tissue gray tones.
   e. The spinous processes should be seen in the center of the lumbar vertebrae.
   f. The ribs and pelvis should be equidistant to the edge of the image receptor on both sides.

Exercise 2: Contrast Studies for the Gallbladder

Instructions: This exercise pertains to radiographic demonstrations of the gallbladder using a contrast medium. Fill in missing words, provide a short answer, or choose true or false (explaining any statement you believe to be false) for each item.

1. Radiographic visualization of the gallbladder after the introduction of a contrast medium is termed

   Cholecystography.

2. The most common method by which a contrast medium is introduced into a patient for cholecystography is the

   Oral method.

3. The commonly used acronym for oral cholecystography is

   OCG.

4. An oral cholecystopaque is absorbed through the intestines

   and transported to the liver by the _Portal_ vein.

5. Define the following terms:

   a. Cholelithiasis: _The presence of calculi in_
   _GB_

   b. Choledocholithiasis: _Calculi in CBD_

   c. Cholecystitis: _Acute or chronic inflammation_
   _of GB_

   d. Biliary stenosis: _A narrowing or occlusion of_
   the CBD

6. The most common pathologic reason for performing oral cholecystography (OCG) is to demonstrate

   gallstones.

7. List six topics that should be included in written instructions given to patients preparing for OCG.

   1. Prelim prep of GI tract
   2. Prelim. diet
   3. Exact time to swallow pills
   4. Avoidance of laxatives
   5. Avoidance of food after swallowing pills
   6. Time to report for exam.

8. After a patient arrives in the radiography department for an OCG examination, why is it important to determine whether the patient experienced vomiting or diarrhea after ingesting the oral cholecystopaque tablets?

   - Vomiting / Diarrhea may have caused contrast to be expelled

9. Why should patients be scheduled for OCG examinations in the early part of the morning?

   - Prolonged fasting can cause ↑ gas, block GB visualization

10. What two purposes may be served by performing a general survey scout radiograph of the patient before preparation for OCG examinations?

    - ✓ if intestinal tract is clean
    - Contrast may obscure gallstones.

11. If the use of a laxative is part of the preparation for an OCG examination, why should the patient be instructed not to use a laxative less than 24 hours before swallowing the oral cholecystopaque tablets?

—To allow irritation of the intestinal mucosa to subside

12. After consuming the oral cholecystopaque tablets but before arriving in the radiography department for the scheduled OCG examination, what food or drink is the patient allowed to consume?

only H_2O

13. What imaging modality is often used to complement an OCG examination if gallbladder images fail to provide a diagnosis?

— ultrasonography

14. True or False. Pure cholesterol gallstones appear as negative filling defects within the opacified bile.

15. True or False. Gallstones containing calcium can often be seen on plain radiography before the introduction of a contrast medium.

Items 16 through 31 pertain to the *PA projection.* Examine Fig. 16-10 as you answer the following items.

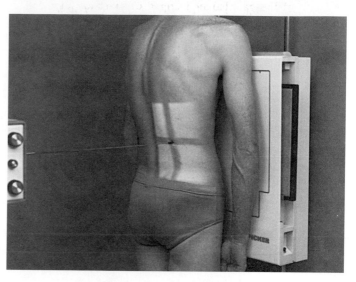

Figure 16-10 PA gallbladder, upright position.

16. True or False. The PA projection can be performed with the patient either in the prone position or upright.

17. True or False. The left side of the patient should be centered to the midline of the table.

18. Which focal spot size—large or small—should be used for radiography of the gallbladder?

— small

19. What kVp range should be used to produce maximum soft tissue differentiation?

70-80

20. What procedure should be performed to prevent pendulous breasts of female patients from superimposing the gallbladder?

    — Spread breasts superiorly & laterally to clear GB

21. With the patient in the prone position, why should the left cheek (rather than the right cheek) rest on a pillow?

    — Rotate vertebrae slightly to left

22. What can be done to the lower limbs to relieve pressure on the toes when the patient is prone?

    Elevate Ankles

23. At what point during patient breathing should the exposure be made?

    After suspension of Expiration.

24. How much time should elapse after the patient suspends respiration before the exposure is made? Explain why.

    2 seconds

25. Examine the radiographs in Figs. 16-11 and 16-12 and answer the questions that follow.

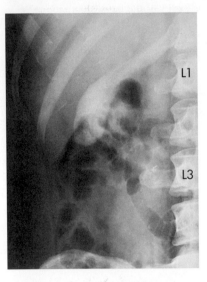

Figure 16-11 Gallbladder radiograph.

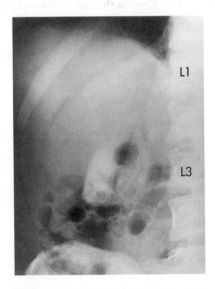

Figure 16-12 Gallbladder radiograph.

a. Which radiograph was exposed after the patient suspended respiration after expiration?

    16-11

b. Which radiograph should be marked to indicate the specific phase of respiration when the exposure was made?

    16-12

26. What procedure should be performed for a subsequent PA projection radiograph with the patient in the prone position if the first PA projection radiograph demonstrates the gallbladder superimposed with rib shadows?

    —Make exposure after pt. suspends respiration after inspiration.

27. Identify the body habitus type—sthenic, asthenic, or hypersthenic—for which each of the following central ray centering levels is used.

    a. 9th costal cartilage: _____ Sthenic _____

    b. 2 inches (5 cm) above the 9th costal cartilage:

       _____ Hypersthenic _____

    c. 2 inches (5 cm) below the 9th costal cartilage:

       _____ Asthenic _____

28. Is the centering point for the patient who has been moved to the standing position from the prone position relatively higher or lower?

    Lower

29. How much does the gallbladder's position shift when a prone patient is moved to the upright position?

    2-4"

30. When the patient is positioned in the upright position, where should gallstones that are heavier than bile be demonstrated within the gallbladder?

    — c̄ fundic portion

31. Listed following are statements pertaining to the prone and upright positions. In the space provided, write *P* if the statement pertains to the prone position or *U* if the statement pertains to the upright position.

    U a. This position can show different layers of gallstones.
    U b. This position best demonstrates mobility of the gallbladder.
    P c. This position produces a foreshortened image of the gallbladder.
    U d. This position usually projects a more vertical image of a gallbladder.
    U e. Radiographs of this position should be marked to indicate the position of the patient.
    P f. This position produces an irregular circular or triangular image of the gallbladder.
    U g. This position is best for demonstrating many gallstones that are too small to be seen individually.
    P h. This position generally requires higher localization centering than the other PA projection.

Items 32 through 42 pertain to the *PA oblique projection (left anterior oblique [LAO] position)* and the *lateral projection (right lateral position)*. Examine Figs. 16-13 and 16-14 as you answer the following items.

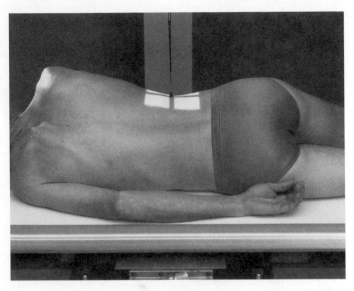

Figure 16-13 PA oblique gallbladder, LAO position.

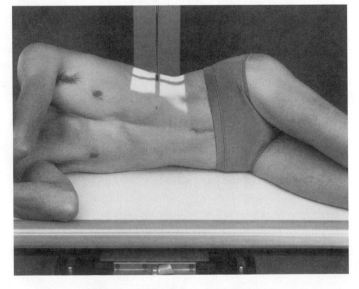

Figure 16-14 Right lateral gallbladder.

32. True or *False* The patient should be upright when positioning for the PA oblique, LAO position.

33. *True* or False. The right side of the patient should be elevated away from the table when positioning for the PA oblique, LAO position.

34. The PA oblique projection, LAO position, is particularly effective in separating the shadow of the gallbladder from

the _____vertebral column_____.

35. How many degrees should the patient be rotated from the prone position for the PA oblique projection, LAO position?

15°-40°

36. List three factors that affect the degree of rotation when positioning the patient for the PA oblique projection, LAO position.

1. The location of GB c̄ ref. to vert. column

2. Angulation of the long Axis of the GB

3. Whether rt. colic flexure is clear or obscures GB

37. Which type of patient—thin or large—requires more rotation when positioning for the PA oblique, LAO position?

Thin

38. Why is the right lateral position preferred over the left lateral position when the lateral projection is performed?

A rt. LAT places GB closer to film

39. The right lateral projection is sometimes used to differentiate gallstones from _____kidney_____ stones.

40. The exposure should be made after the patient has suspended respiration after _____ _EXP._ _____.

41. The right lateral position is useful for separating the shadows of the gallbladder and the vertebrae for patients who are exceptionally _____ _Thin_ _____ (large or thin).

42. Cholecystograms should demonstrate the gallbladder and surrounding structures in _____ _Short Scale_ _____ (long-scale or short-scale) contrast.

Items 43 through 50 pertain to the *AP projection (right lateral decubitus position)*. Examine Fig. 16-15 as you answer the following items.

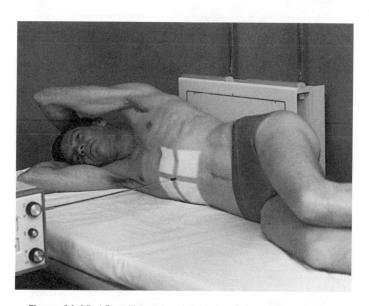

Figure 16-15 AP gallbladder, right lateral decubitus position.

43. Why should the patient be elevated 2 to 3 inches (5 to 7.6 cm) on a suitable radiolucent support?
    a. To demonstrate vertebral bodies
    b. To ensure that the diaphragm is included in the image
    (c.) To center the gallbladder region to the image receptor

44. Which term best describes how the central ray should be directed?
    a. Angled
    b. Vertically
    (c.) Horizontally

45. One advantage of this position is that the gallbladder should gravitate toward the _____ _right_ _____ (right or left) side.

46. With reference to adjacent gas-containing loops of the intestine, the gallbladder should lie _____ _below_ _____ (above or below) gas shadows.

47. Which contrast scale—long or short—should be used to best demonstrate the gallbladder?

    Short

48. In addition to a side marker, what other marker should be seen on the radiograph?

    —Decubitus

49. (True) or False. The right lateral decubitus position is used for stratification studies of the low-placed gallbladder.

50. True or (False). The left lateral decubitus position should be used for demonstrating gallstones if the patient is unable to stand.

Exercise 3: Identifying Gallbladder Radiographs

Instructions: Examine the images of gallbladders in Figs.16-16 through 16-19. Based on the appearance or the location of each gallbladder relative to its surrounding structures, identify in which position the patient was most likely placed for the exposure: PA (prone), PA (upright), left anterior oblique (LAO), or right lateral decubitus.

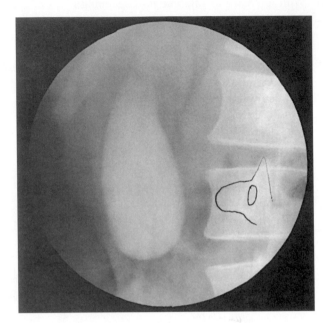

Figure 16-16 Gallbladder radiograph.

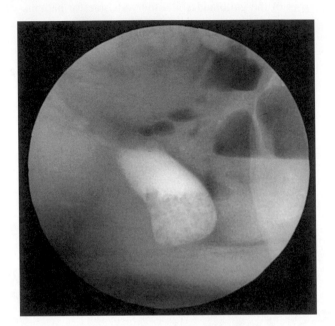

Figure 16-17 Gallbladder radiograph.

1. Fig. 16-16: _____ LAO _____

2. Fig. 16-17: _____ RT. LAT Decl _____

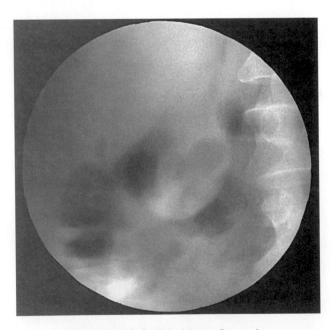

Figure 16-18 Gallbladder radiograph.

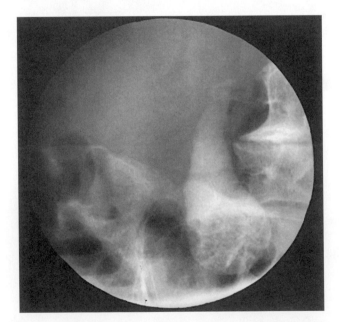

Figure 16-19 Gallbladder radiograph.

3. Fig. 16-18: _____ PA Prone _____

4. Fig. 16-19: _____ PA UPRT. _____

Self-Test: Abdomen, Liver, Spleen, and Biliary Tract

Instructions: Answer the following questions by selecting the best choice.

1. Which organ produces bile?
   a. Liver
   b. Spleen
   c. Pancreas
   d. Gallbladder

2. Which body function does the pancreas perform?
   a. Filtration of blood
   b. Production of bile
   c. Production of lymphocytes
   d. Production of digestive juices

3. Which organ stores and concentrates bile?
   a. Liver
   b. Spleen
   c. Pancreas
   d. Gallbladder

4. Which substance activates the muscular contraction of the gallbladder?
   a. Bile
   b. Cholecystokinin
   c. Pancreatic juices
   d. Cholecystolithiasis

5. The spleen is part of which body system?
   a. Urinary
   b. Digestive
   c. Endocrine
   d. Lymphatic

6. In which organ are clusters of islet cells found?
   a. Liver
   b. Spleen
   c. Pancreas
   d. Gallbladder

7. How many major lobes does the liver have?
   a. One
   b. Two
   c. Three
   d. Four

8. Which structure forms the mesentery and omenta folds?
   a. Liver
   b. Pancreas
   c. Gallbladder
   d. Peritoneum

9. Which organ's blood is supplied by the portal vein?
   a. Liver
   b. Spleen
   c. Pancreas
   d. Gallbladder

10. Which duct is formed by the merging of the right and left hepatic ducts?
    a. Cystic
    b. Pancreatic
    c. Common bile
    d. Common hepatic

11. Which duct is formed by the union of the cystic duct with the common hepatic duct?
    a. Pancreatic
    b. Left hepatic
    c. Right hepatic
    d. Common bile

12. Where do the pancreatic and common bile ducts terminate?
    a. Ileum
    b. Duodenum
    c. Gallbladder
    d. Large intestine

13. Which duct connects the gallbladder to the common hepatic duct?
    a. Cystic
    b. Pancreatic
    c. Right hepatic
    d. Common bile

14. Which three projections usually comprise the acute abdomen series for ambulatory patients?
    a. Supine KUB, AP upright abdomen, and PA chest
    b. Supine KUB, right lateral decubitus abdomen, and PA chest
    c. Left lateral decubitus abdomen, dorsal decubitus abdomen, and PA chest
    d. Right lateral decubitus abdomen, left lateral decubitus abdomen, and dorsal decubitus abdomen

15. To which level of the patient should the IR be centered for the KUB?
    a. T10 vertebral body
    b. L3 vertebral body
    c. 2 inches (5 cm) above the iliac crests
    d. Iliac crests

16. For the AP upright abdomen radiograph of an adult of average size, why should the IR be slightly raised above the centering level used for the supine KUB radiograph?

    a. To include the bladder
    b. To include the diaphragm
    c. To visualize gallstones
    d. To visualize kidney stones

17. For the KUB radiograph, when should respiration be suspended, and what effect will that have on the patient?

    a. On full expiration; elevate the diaphragm
    b. On full expiration; depress the diaphragm
    c. On full inspiration; elevate the diaphragm
    d. On full inspiration; depress the diaphragm

18. Why is it desirable to include the diaphragm in the upright abdomen radiograph?

    a. To demonstrate free air in the abdomen
    b. To demonstrate fluid levels in the thorax
    c. To demonstrate fluid levels in the abdomen
    d. To demonstrate calculi in the gallbladder and kidneys

19. Which of the following guidelines is *not* necessary to follow when deciding whether to use gonadal shielding for the KUB radiograph?

    a. The patient has reasonable reproductive potential.
    b. The gonads lie within 2 inches (5 cm) of the primary beam.
    c. The purpose for performing the examination is not compromised.
    d. The permission to use gonadal shielding is granted by the patient.

20. Which projection should be used to demonstrate free air within the abdominal cavity when the patient is unable to stand for an upright abdomen radiograph?

    a. AP projection with the patient supine
    b. Lateral projection, dorsal decubitus position
    c. AP projection, left lateral decubitus position
    d. AP projection, right lateral decubitus position

21. Which projection does not demonstrate free air levels within the abdomen?

    a. AP projection with the patient supine
    b. AP projection with the patient upright
    c. Lateral projection, dorsal decubitus position
    d. AP projection, left lateral decubitus position

22. What is the major advantage of the PA projection of the abdomen over the AP projection of the abdomen?

    a. The PA projection reduces the exposure dose to the gonads.
    b. The PA projection magnifies gallstones for better visualization.
    c. The PA projection demonstrates the pubic rami below the urinary bladder.
    d. The PA projection reduces the object-to-image receptor distance of the kidneys.

23. Which radiographic position of the abdomen requires that the patient be placed in the lateral recumbent position on his or her left side and that the central ray be directed along the midsagittal plane, entering the anterior surface of the patient's abdomen at the level of the iliac crests?

    a. Dorsal decubitus
    b. Ventral decubitus
    c. Left lateral decubitus
    d. Right lateral decubitus

24. Which radiographic position of the abdomen requires that the patient be supine and that the central ray be directed to a lateral side of the patient, entering slightly anterior to the midcoronal plane?

    a. Dorsal decubitus
    b. Ventral decubitus
    c. Left lateral decubitus
    d. Right lateral decubitus

25. Which radiographic position of the abdomen requires that the patient be placed in the lateral recumbent position on his or her left side, that the IR be placed under the patient and centered to the abdomen at the level of the iliac crests, and that the central ray be directed to enter the right side of the patient slightly anterior to the midcoronal plane?

    a. Left lateral
    b. Right lateral
    c. Left lateral decubitus
    d. Right lateral decubitus

26. The lateral projection with the patient placed in the dorsal decubitus position, the left lateral projection, and the left lateral decubitus position of the abdomen all require which of the following?

    a. The central ray should enter the left side of the patient.
    b. The patient should suspend respiration after expiration.
    c. The patient should suspend respiration after inspiration.
    d. The central ray should enter the anterior side of the abdomen.

27. For the lateral projection with the patient placed in the dorsal decubitus position, where should the central ray enter the patient?

    a. 2 inches (5 cm) anterior to the midcoronal plane at the level of the iliac crests
    b. 2 inches (5 cm) anterior to the midcoronal plane and 2 inches above the level of the iliac crests
    c. 2 inches (5 cm) posterior to the midcoronal plane at the level of the iliac crests
    d. 2 inches (5 cm) posterior to the midcoronal plane and 2 inches above the level of the iliac crests

28. For the lateral projection with the patient placed in the dorsal decubitus position, which procedure should be performed to ensure that the entire abdomen is included on the radiograph?

    a. Use support cushions to elevate the patient.
    b. Center the IR to the level of the xiphoid process.
    c. Center the IR to the anterior surface of the abdomen.
    d. Direct the central ray to a point 2 inches (5 cm) below the iliac crests.

29. Which structures should be examined to see whether the patient was rotated for a lateral projection of the abdomen?

    a. Pelvis and lumbar vertebrae
    b. Pelvis and thoracic vertebrae
    c. Diaphragm and lumbar vertebrae
    d. Diaphragm and thoracic vertebrae

30. Which imaging procedure should be part of the OCG examination?

    a. Use long exposure times and long-scale contrast.
    b. Use long exposure times and short-scale contrast.
    c. Use short exposure times and long-scale contrast.
    d. Use short exposure times and short-scale contrast.

31. For OCG procedures, when should respiration be suspended, and what effect will this have on the position of the gallbladder?

    a. On full inspiration; depress the gallbladder
    b. On full inspiration; elevate the gallbladder
    c. On full expiration; depress the gallbladder
    d. On full expiration; elevate the gallbladder

32. Which procedure should be performed when the patient is rotated from a prone position to the LAO position for an OCG examination?

    a. Make the exposure after full inspiration.
    b. Center the IR to the left side of the patient.
    c. Center the IR to the level of the diaphragm.
    d. Place a radiolucent foam wedge under the abdomen.

33. For an OCG examination of a patient of average build, where should the IR be centered?

    a. At the level of the 9th rib on the left side
    b. At the level of the 9th rib on the right side
    c. At the level of the 12th rib on the left side
    d. At the level of the 12th rib on the right side

34. Compared to IR placement for a patient of average build, how should the IR be moved for an OCG examination of a hypersthenic patient?

    a. Lower
    b. Higher
    c. To the left of the vertebral column
    d. More to the lateral side of the right side of the abdomen

35. Which procedure should be performed for a subsequent PA projection radiograph when the initial PA projection radiograph demonstrates the shadow of the gallbladder superimposed by ribs?

    a. Make the exposure after full inspiration.
    b. Use radiolucent cushions to elevate the patient.
    c. Direct the central ray caudally 10 to 15 degrees.
    d. Place the patient in the Trendelenburg position.

36. Which procedure most effectively separates the shadows of the gallbladder and vertebrae?

    a. Make the exposure after full inspiration.
    b. Rotate the patient into an oblique position.
    c. Place the patient in the Trendelenburg position.
    d. Position the patient for a dorsal decubitus projection.

37. Which projection best demonstrates the stratification of gallstones?

    a. AP projection with the patient supine
    b. PA projection with the patient prone
    c. AP projection, right lateral decubitus position
    d. PA oblique projection (right anterior oblique [RAO] position) with the patient recumbent

38. Which procedure best demonstrates a gallbladder that is situated in the iliac fossa?

    a. Place the patient in the prone position.
    b. Place the patient in the supine position.
    c. Place the patient in the upright position.
    d. Make the exposure after full inspiration.

39. Why should patients be scheduled for OCG examinations in the early morning?

    a. Prolonged fasting causes the formation of gas.
    b. Scheduling conflicts with fluoroscopy are prevented.
    c. Continual production of bile dilutes the contrast medium.
    d. A gallbladder can only store contrast medium for 8 hours.

40. Which projection places the gallbladder closest to the IR?

    a. PA projection
    b. AP projection
    c. PA oblique projection (LAO position) with the patient upright
    d. AP oblique projection (left posterior oblique [LPO] position) with the patient recumbent

41. Which procedure should not be performed as part of patient preparation for the OCG examination?

    a. Administer a cleansing enema to prepare the intestinal tract.
    b. Instruct the patient to consume only water after swallowing oral contrast medium.
    c. Instruct the patient to take laxatives within 24 hours before swallowing oral contrast medium.
    d. Give the patient a fat-free evening meal to consume shortly before swallowing oral contrast medium.

42. Which diagnostic modality is most often used when an OCG examination does not adequately demonstrate a gallbladder?

    a. Sonography
    b. Nuclear medicine
    c. Computed tomography
    d. Magnetic resonance imaging

43. Which projection produces a foreshortened image of the gallbladder?

    a. Right lateral projection
    b. PA projection with the patient prone
    c. PA projection with the patient upright
    d. PA oblique projection (LAO position) with the patient upright

44. Which of the following projections does not increase the separation of the gallbladder shadow from the vertebrae?

    a. PA projection
    b. AP projection, right lateral decubitus position
    c. PA oblique projection (LAO position) with the patient upright
    d. PA oblique projection (LAO position) with the patient recumbent

45. Which procedure should be performed for the left PA oblique projection that is part of an OCG examination?

    a. Make the exposure after full inspiration.
    b. Rotate thin patients more than large patients.
    c. Rotate large patients more than thin patients.
    d. Center the image receptor to the left upper quadrant.

46. Which procedure should be performed when using the right lateral decubitus position that is part of an OCG examination?

    a. Place the patient on a radiolucent cushion.
    b. Center the IR to the level of the iliac crests.
    c. Use a marker to indicate that the right side of the patient is the "up" side.
    d. Place the patient in the lateral recumbent position with the left side down.

47. What is an advantage to using the right lateral decubitus position for demonstration of the gallbladder?

    a. This position enables the gallbladder to be separated from the liver.
    b. This position enables the stomach to provide a homogeneous background density.
    c. This position enables the gallbladder to gravitate toward the dependent left side of the abdomen.
    d. This position enables the gallbladder to gravitate toward the dependent right side of the abdomen.

48. Which two projections best visualize the stratification of gallstones?

    a. AP supine KUB and prone PA projections
    b. AP supine KUB and upright PA projections
    c. AP (right lateral decubitus position) and prone PA projections
    d. AP (right lateral decubitus position) and upright PA projections

49. Which projection is generally not used as part of the OCG examination?

    a. PA projection
    b. PA oblique projection (LAO position)
    c. AP projection, right lateral decubitus position
    d. Lateral projection, dorsal decubitus position

50. Which projection of the gallbladder can be performed only with a horizontally directed central ray?

    a. PA projection
    b. Right lateral projection
    c. PA oblique projection (LAO position)
    d. AP projection, right lateral decubitus position

CHAPTER 17

Digestive System: Alimentary Canal

SECTION 1

Anatomy of the Alimentary Canal

Exercise 1

Instructions: This exercise pertains to the digestive system. Identify structures for each question.

1. Identify each lettered structure shown in Fig. 17-1.

A. _____

B. _____

C. _____

D. _____

E. _____

F. _____

G. _____

H. _____

I. _____

J. _____

K. _____

L. _____

M. _____

N. _____

O. _____

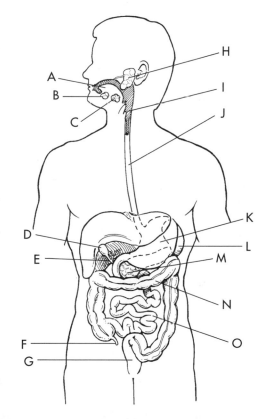

Figure 17-1 The alimentary canal and its accessory organs.

2. Identify each lettered structure shown in Fig. 17-2.

A. _____

B. _____

C. _____

D. _____

E. _____

F. _____

G. _____

H. _____

I. _____

J. _____

K. _____

L. _____

3. Identify each lettered structure shown in Fig. 17-3.

A. _____

B. _____

C. _____

D. _____

E. _____

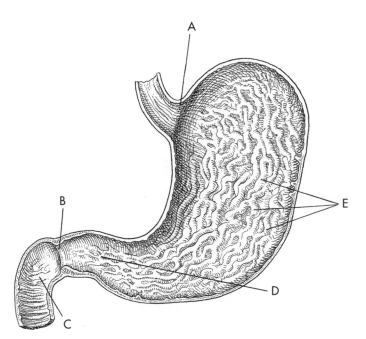

Figure 17-3 Section of the stomach showing rugae.

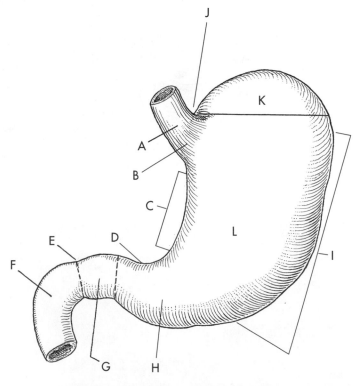

Figure 17-2 Anterior surface of the stomach.

4. Identify each lettered structure shown in Fig. 17-4.

A. _____

B. _____

C. _____

D. _____

E. _____

F. _____

G. _____

H. _____

I. _____

J. _____

K. _____

5. Identify each lettered structure shown in Fig. 17-5.

A. _____

B. _____

C. _____

D. _____

E. _____

F. _____

G. _____

H. _____

I. _____

J. _____

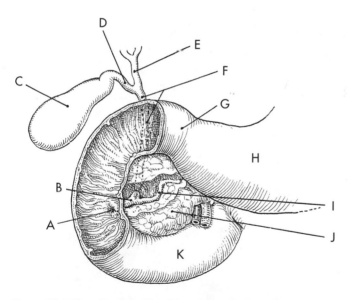

Figure 17-4 The duodenal loop in relation to the biliary and pancreatic ducts.

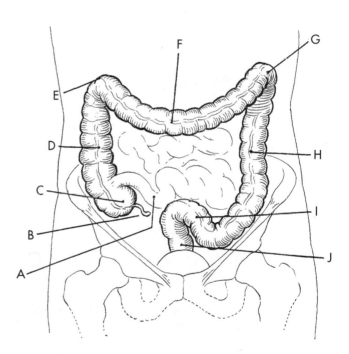

Figure 17-5 Anterior aspect of the large bowel.

6. Identify each lettered structure shown in Fig. 17-6.

A. _____

B. _____

C. _____

D. _____

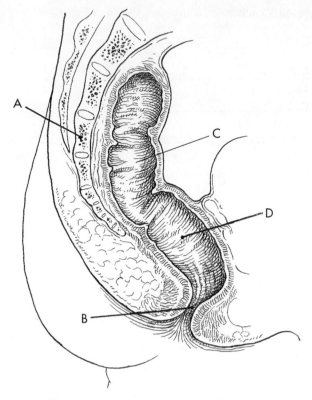

Figure 17-6 Sagittal section showing the anal canal and rectum.

Exercise 2

Instructions: Use the following clues to complete the crossword puzzle. All answers refer to the alimentary canal.

ACROSS

1. Stores bile
5. Gastric folds
8. Attached to cecum
10. Terminates alimentary canal
11. Widest part of alimentary canal
15. Contraction waves
18. Proximal part of small bowel
19. Left colic flexure
22. Between cecum and right colic flexure

23. Average body build
24. Precedes anal canal

DOWN

2. Digestive juice
3. Musculomembranous tube
4. Upper part of stomach
6. Lower than sthenic
7. Proximal part of large intestine

9. Precedes esophagus
12. Large body build
13. Middle part of small bowel
14. Very slender body build
16. Intestinal bend
17. Between left colic flexure and sigmoid
20. Produces bile
21. Distal part of small bowel

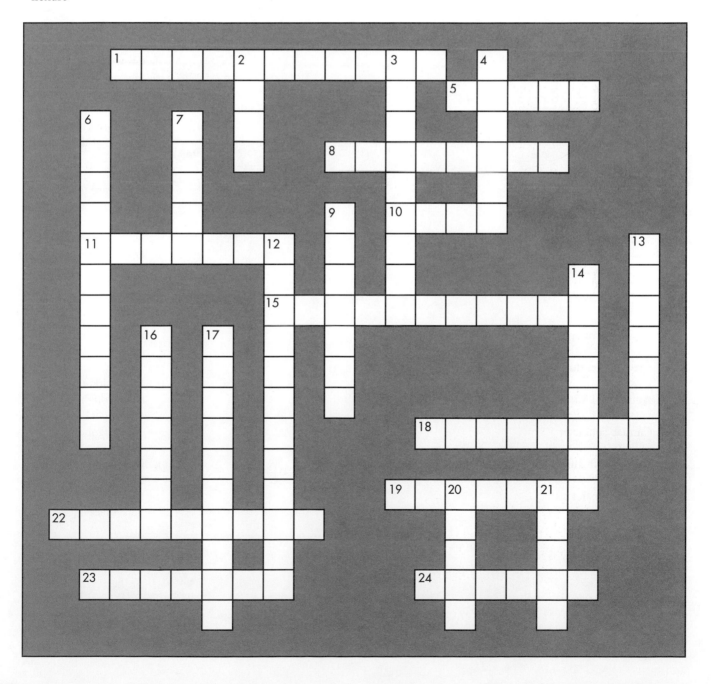

Exercise 3

Instructions: Match the structures or portions of organs found in the alimentary canal from the list in Column A with the major organs to which they most closely relate as listed in Column B.

Column A

_____ 1. Bulb

_____ 2. Body

_____ 3. Rugae

_____ 4. Ileum

_____ 5. Cecum

_____ 6. Rectum

_____ 7. Fundus

_____ 8. Pylorus

_____ 9. Sigmoid

_____ 10. Jejunum

_____ 11. Duodenum

_____ 12. Transverse

_____ 13. Ascending

_____ 14. Descending

_____ 15. Lesser curvature

_____ 16. Greater curvature

_____ 17. Ampulla of Vater

_____ 18. Cardiac sphincter

_____ 19. Left colic flexure

_____ 20. Right colic flexure

Column B

a. Stomach

b. Small intestine

c. Large intestine

Exercise 4.

Instructions: Match the pathology terms in Column A with the appropriate definition in Column B. Not all choices from Column B should be selected.

Column A

_____ 1. Ulcer

_____ 2. Polyp

_____ 3. Reflux

_____ 4. Colitis

_____ 5. Gastritis

_____ 6. Volvulus

_____ 7. Diverticulum

_____ 8. Diverticulosis

_____ 9. Intussusception

_____ 10. Inguinal hernia

Column B

a. Inflammation of the colon

b. Twisting of a bowel loop on itself

c. Protrusion of the bowel into the groin

d. Inflammation of the lining of the stomach

e. Growth or mass protruding from a mucous membrane

f. Depressed lesion of the surface of the alimentary canal

g. Backward flow of the stomach contents into the esophagus

h. Diverticula in the colon without inflammation or symptoms

i. Prolapse of a portion of the bowel into the lumen of an adjacent part

j. Protrusion of the stomach through the esophageal hiatus of the diaphragm

k. Pouch created by the herniation of the mucous membrane through the muscular coat

Exercise 5

Instructions: This exercise pertains to the alimentary canal and its related organs. Fill in missing words or provide a short answer for each question.

1. The musculomembranous passage that extends from the pharynx to the stomach is the _____.

2. The expanded part of the distal end of the esophagus is the _____ _____.

3. The opening into the stomach through which food and liquids pass is the _____ _____.

4. The organ in which gastric digestion begins is the _____.

5. The gastric folds of the stomach are the _____.

6. The border of the stomach with the lesser curvature is the _____ border.

7. The lesser curvature extends from the esophagogastric junction to the _____.

8. The left and inferior borders of the stomach are the _____ _____.

9. Figure 17-7 shows four diagrams, each representing a different body habitus. Indicate in the blanks provided which of the following body habitus type each diagram represents: sthenic, asthenic, hyposthenic, or hypersthenic.

a. Diagram A: _____

b. Diagram B: _____

c. Diagram C: _____

d. Diagram D: _____

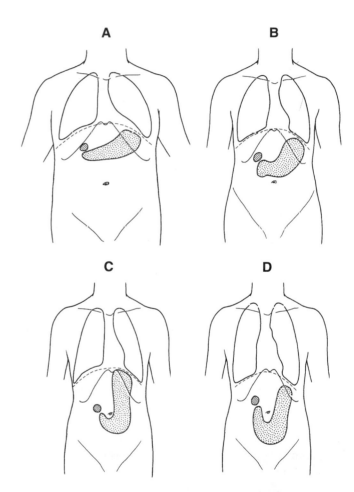

Figure 17-7 The four types of body habitus.

10. Name the four parts of the stomach.

11. The part of the stomach immediately surrounding the esophageal opening is the _____.

12. The most superior part of the stomach is the _____.

13. The most inferior part of the stomach is the _____ portion.

14. The opening between the stomach and the small intestine is the _____.

15. The three parts of the small intestine are the _____, _____, and _____.

16. The proximal part of the small intestine is the _____.

17. The radiographically significant first segment of the proximal part of the small intestine is the _____ _____.

18. The small intestine terminates at the _____ _____.

19. The common bile and the pancreatic ducts empty into the _____.

20. The middle part of the small intestine is the _____.

21. The distal part of the small intestine is the _____.

22. The shortest part the small intestine is the _____; the longest part is the _____.

23. The longer of the two intestines is the _____ intestine.

24. The passage from the small intestine to the large intestine is the _____ _____.

25. The proximal part of the large intestine is the _____.

26. The veriform appendix attaches to the large intestine at the _____.

27. Located between the ascending colon and the transverse colon is the _____ flexure.

28. The part of the colon that extends from the cecum to the right colic flexure is the _____ colon.

29. The part of the colon that extends between the two flexures is the _____ colon.

30. Located between the transverse colon and the descending colon is the _____ flexure.

31. The part of the colon that extends inferiorly from the left colic flexure is the _____ colon.

32. The sigmoid colon is located between the two parts of the large intestine known as the _____ and the _____.

33. The sigmoid colon terminates in the _____.

34. The part of the large intestine that extends between the rectum and the anus is the _____.

35. The external opening at the terminal end of the anal canal is the _____.

SECTION 2

Positioning of the Alimentary Canal

Exercise 1: Positioning for the Esophagus

Instructions: The esophagus can be radiographically examined after a contrast medium has been introduced. This exercise pertains to procedures used to obtain the required radiographs of the esophagus. Fill in missing words, provide a short answer, or choose true or false (explaining any statement you believe to be false) for each item.

1. List the projections that comprise the typical esophageal study.

   -AP /PA

   - RAO /LPO

   - LAT. Projection

2. What two types of contrast media are used for double-contrast esophageal studies?

   - High Density Barium

   CO₂ Crystals

3. Why is the left PA oblique projection, left anterior oblique (LAO) position, not included in the typical esophageal study?

   - Superimposition of vertebrae c̄ esophagus

4. When demonstrating the entire esophagus, to what level of the patient should the image receptor (IR) be centered?

   T₅-T₆

   top of
   - IR @ level of mouth

5. What two oblique positions can be used to demonstrate the entire esophagus effectively?

   RAO /LPO

6. Why is the recumbent right anterior oblique (RAO) position preferred over the upright position?

   Allows complete filling of esophagus

7. For anteroposterior (AP) or posteroanterior (PA) projections, how is it determined that the selection of exposure factors was acceptable?

   - Esophagus adequately demonstrated through superimposed thoracic vertebrae.

8. In relation to the surrounding structures, where should the esophagus appear in images with the patient in the RAO position?

   - To left of vert. column, between thoracic vertebrae & heart

9. In radiographs of a contrast-filled esophagus with the patient in the RAO position, how does the esophagus appear in relation to the surrounding structures when rotation of the patient was insufficient?

   - Partially obscured by thoracic vertebrae.

10. In the lateral projection radiograph, what structures are used to determine whether the patient was rotated? How should these structures appear?

Post. ribs Superimposed

11. For radiographs with the patient in the RAO position, the patient should be rotated approximately __*35*__ to __*40*__ degrees.

12. The esophagus should be clearly seen from the lower neck to the __*Cardiac orifice*__ _____.

13. (True) or False. Single-contrast and double-contrast studies can be used to demonstrate the esophagus.

14. (True) or False. A barium sulfate mixture is the preferred contrast medium for esophagrams.

15. True or (False). The most important requirement for the contrast medium is that the weight per volume should be rated greater than 50%. *(30% – 50%)*

Exercise 2: The Gastrointestinal Series

Instructions: One of the more commonly performed studies employing contrast media is the gastrointestinal (GI) series. This exercise pertains to gastrointestinal studies. Identify structures, fill in missing words, provide a short answer, select from a list, or choose true or false (explaining any statement you believe to be false) for each item.

Items 1 through 20 pertain to upper gastrointestinal (UGI) examination procedures.

1. What acronym refers to the upper gastrointestinal series?

UGI

2. As part of patient preparation, why should the patient maintain a soft, low-residue diet for two days?

↓ gas / fecal matter

3. How can the UGI study be affected if the patient smokes cigarettes shortly before the examination?

— gastric secretions. would dilute barium

4. What type of radiopaque contrast medium usually is used in routine UGI studies?

Barium product of 30% – 50%
weight / volume concentration

5. List the two general GI examination procedures routinely used to examine the stomach.

Single Contrast exam & double contrast exam

6. What is the range of weight per volume concentration for the barium sulfate suspension usually used for single-contrast examinations?

    30% - 50%

7. List two advantages of performing the double-contrast examination.

    1) Small lesions easily demonstrated

    2) mucosal lining of stomach clearly visualized

8. What are the two types of contrast media used in double-contrast procedures?

    High density BaSO₄ & gas producing substance.

9. True or ~~False~~. Both the single-contrast and double-contrast procedures should begin with the patient in the lateral recumbent position.   Pt. ↑

10. True or ~~False~~. After the patient consumes the barium sulfate suspension for a double-contrast examination, all radiographs should be performed with the patient in the upright position.   pt recumbent

11. ~~True~~ or False. The barium sulfate suspension used for double-contrast examinations should have a higher weight per volume ratio than the barium sulfate suspension used for single-contrast examinations.

12. Why should patients undergoing double-contrast examinations turn from side-to-side or roll over a few times during the procedure?

    Coat mucosal lining of stomach.

13. During double-contrast examinations, what instructions should be given to the patient after the patient swallows the carbon dioxide crystals or tablets to ensure a double-contrast effect?

    - Pt should not belch

14. What is the purpose of using glucagon during the double-contrast examination?

    - Relax gastric tract, enabling gastric structure to expand & be more easily demonstrated.

15. What is a biphasic GI examination?

    1ˢᵗ examined c̄ double contrast
    ↓
    low weight per volume BaSO₄ administered in single - contrast

16. Which method of examination—the single-contrast or double-contrast—is performed first as part of a biphasic examination?

    double contrast

17. What are the two methods of performing hypotonic duodenography?

    c̄ / s̄ intubation

18. (True) or False. Hypotonic duodenography originally required that the contrast medium be introduced directly through a tube placed into the duodenum.

19. (True) or False. The tubeless hypotonic duodenography examination is performed after a drug has temporarily paralyzed the duodenum.

20. (True) or False. Other imaging modalities such as sonography and computed tomography have largely replaced hypotonic duodenography.

Items 21 through 31 pertain to the *PA projection*. Examine Fig. 17-8 as you answer the following items.

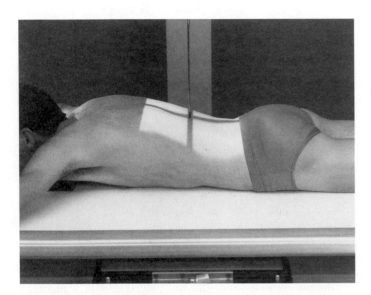

Figure 17-8 PA stomach and duodenum.

21. True or (False.) Routine radiographs of the stomach and duodenum should be made with the patient in the upright position. *Pt· Recumbent*

22. (True) or False. The PA projection with the patient in the prone position demonstrates the contour of the barium-filled stomach and duodenal bulb.

23. (True) or False. The PA projection with the patient in the upright position shows the size, shape, and relative position of the barium-filled stomach.

24. True or (False.) A compression band may be placed across the patient's abdomen to immobilize the patient and reduce involuntary movement of the viscera. *no may cause Artifact.*

25. How should the prone position of the patient be adjusted to prevent the full weight of the abdomen from causing the stomach and duodenum to press against the vertebral column?

Pts weight supported by cushion placed under thorax & pelvis.

26. How should the patient's position be adjusted to center the stomach over the midline of the table?

- Midline of grid
- Sagittal plane passing ½ way between vert. column & Lt. lat. border of Abd.

27. When performing the PA projection on a prone patient, to what level of the patient should the image receptor be centered?

¢ 1-2" above lower rib margin @ L-1- L-2.

28. How should the centering of the IR be adjusted if the patient is repositioned from the prone position to the upright position?

Center IR 3-6" lower.

29. With which body habitus does the greatest visceral movement occur between the prone position and the upright position?

Asthenic

30. What breathing instructions should be given the patient when making the exposure?

Suspend after exp.

31. How and to where should the central ray be directed?

⊥ *to center of IR*

Items 32 through 37 pertain to the *PA oblique projection (RAO position)*. Examine Fig. 17-9 as you answer the following items.

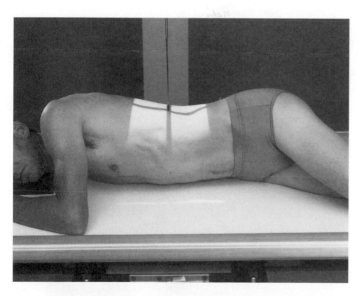

Figure 17-9 PA oblique stomach and duodenum, RAO position.

32. Describe how the patient should be adjusted from the prone position to the RAO position.

Instruct pt. to turn toward Lt, elevate left side, support raised Lt. side c̄ left forearm & flexed Lt. knee.

33. How and to where should the central ray be directed?

⊥ *to center of IR*

34. How many degrees should the patient be rotated from the prone position?
    a. 10 to 15
    b. 20 to 35
    c. 40 to 70

35. Which type of body habitus requires the most rotation?
    a. Sthenic
    b. Hyposthenic
    c. Hypersthenic

36. True or False. For the average patient, the PA oblique projection (RAO position) produces the best image of the pyloric canal and the duodenal bulb filled with barium.

37. True or False. The PA oblique projection (RAO position) radiograph should be exposed when the patient has suspended respiration after full inspiration.

exp.

Items 38 through 45 pertain to the *left AP oblique projection (left posterior oblique [LPO] position)*. Examine Fig. 17-10 as you answer the following items.

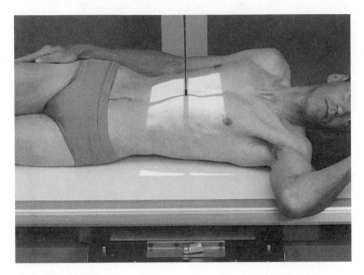

Figure 17-10 AP oblique stomach and duodenum, LPO position.

38. The left AP oblique projection (LPO position) is best performed if the patient is adjusted from the

_____ (supine or prone) position.

39. The side of the patient that should be elevated away from the table is the _____ Rt. _____ (right or left) side.

40. For the left AP oblique projection (LPO position), most patients should be rotated _____ 45 _____ degrees.

41. To what level of the patient should the image receptor be centered?   Midway between xiphoid & lower LAT margin of ribs

42. Where exactly should the CR enter the patient?
Midway between MSP & Lt. LAT. margin of stomach.
– Centered to a level midway between xiphoid & lower LAT. margin of ribs.

43. (True) or False. The left AP oblique projection (LPO position) demonstrates the fundic portion of the stomach filled with barium.

44. True or (False.) The left AP oblique projection (LPO position) demonstrates the pyloric canal and duodenal bulb filled with barium.   Fundus

45. Identify each lettered structure shown in Fig. 17-11.

A. _____ Distal Esophagus _____

B. _____ Fundus _____

C. _____ Body _____

D. _____ Pylorus _____

E. _____ Duodenum. _____

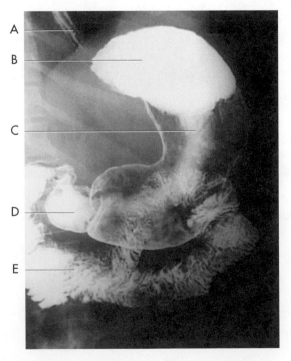

Figure 17-11 AP stomach and duodenum, LPO position.

Items 46 through 53 pertain to the *right lateral projection.* Examine Fig. 17-12 as you answer the following items.

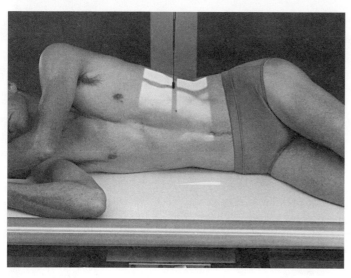

Figure 17-12 Right lateral stomach and duodenum.

46. Which radiographic body position should be used to best demonstrate the duodenal loop and the duodenojejunal junction filled with contrast medium?
    a. Upright RAO position
    b. Recumbent LPO position
    c. Upright left lateral position
    d. Recumbent right lateral position

47. At which vertebral level should the central ray enter the patient if the patient is in the recumbent position?
    a. T10 to T11
    b. L1 to L2
    c. L5 to S1

48. Approximately how many inches above the lower rib margin should the image receptor be centered to the recumbent patient?
    a. 1 to 2
    b. 3 to 4
    c. 5 to 6

49. At which vertebral level should the central ray enter the patient if the patient is moved from the recumbent position to the upright lateral position?
    a. T12
    b. L1
    c. L3
    d. L5

50. When examining right lateral projection radiographs, which osteologic structures should be examined to determine whether the patient was rotated?
    a. Ribs
    b. Vertebrae
    c. Pelvic bones

51. Describe how and to where the central ray should be directed to the IR and the patient.

    - ⊥ to center of IR midway between mid coronal & ant. surface of Abd.

52. Examine Fig. 17-13 and indicate whether the following gastric structures are mostly barium-filled or mostly gas-filled:

a. Stomach fundus: _____ gas filled _____

b. Duodenal bulb: _____ BA " _____

c. Duodenum: _____ Ba " _____

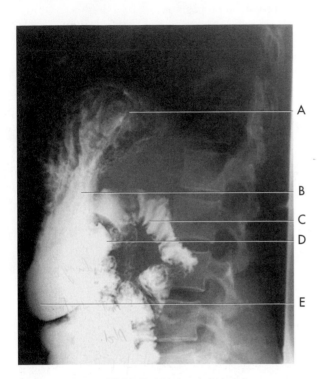

Figure 17-13 Right lateral stomach.

53. Identify each lettered structure shown in Fig. 17-13.

A. _____ Fundus _____

B. _____ Body _____

C. _____ Duodenum _____

D. _____ Duodenal Bulb _____

E. _____ Pyloric portion. _____

Items 54 through 60 pertain to the *AP projection*. Examine Fig. 17-14 as you answer the following items.

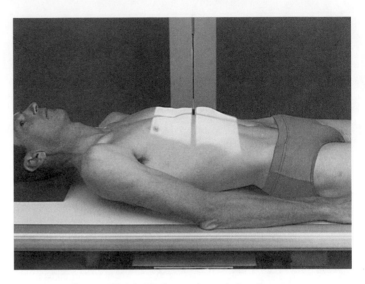

Figure 17-14 AP stomach and duodenum.

54. Which body position should be used?

a. Prone
b. Supine
c. Upright

55. Which procedure should be performed to help demonstrate a diaphragmatic herniation (hiatal hernia)?

a. Tilt the table to Fowler's angulation.
b. Place the patient in the upright position.
c. Tilt the table to the Trendelenburg angulation.
d. Place the patient in the right lateral recumbent position.

56. Describe how the patient should be centered to the grid when using a 35 × 43 cm image receptor.

MSP to midline of grid

57. Describe how the patient should be centered to the grid when using a 30 × 35 cm image receptor.

Saggital plane passing midway between MJP & LAT margin of Lt-Ribs to midline of grid

58. When using the 30 × 35cm image receptor, to what level of the patient should it be centered?

Midway between tip of the xiphoid process & the lower margin of ribs.

59. How should each of the following structures be demonstrated—barium-filled or gas-filled (double-contrast)?

a. Body: _____ gas filled _____

b. Fundus: _____ Ba " _____

c. Pylorus: _____ Gas " _____

d. Duodenal bulb: _____ Gas " _____

60. Identify each lettered structure shown in Fig. 17-15.

A. _____ Fundal _____

B. _____ Body _____

C. _____ Pyloric Portion _____

D. _____ Duodenal Loop, _____

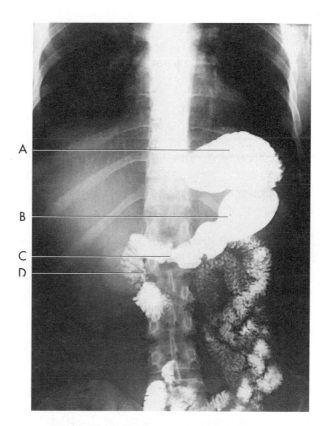

Figure 17-15 AP stomach and duodenum.

Exercise 3: Small Intestine Examination

Instructions: The small intestine can be radiographically examined by more than one method, often after the stomach is examined. This exercise pertains to the small intestine examination, often referred to as the *small bowel series*. Provide a short answer or select the answer from a list for each item.

1. List the three methods by which a barium sulfate mixture can be administered for a small bowel series.

   Oral

   Reflux

   intubation

2. Which small bowel series method is most commonly used?

   a. Oral
   b. Enteroclysis
   c. Complete reflux

3. Select the four instructions from the following list that are usually given to patients preparing for the oral method of performing a small bowel series.

   a. A cleansing enema
   b. No breakfast on the morning of the examination
   c. No evening meal the night before the examination
   d. Swallow laxatives the morning of the examination
   e. Drinking 3 to 4 glasses of water the morning of the examination
   f. Nothing by mouth after the evening meal the night before the examination
   g. A restricted diet (soft, low-residue foods) for up to 2 days before the examination

4. Why is a time marker displayed on each radiograph made during the oral method small bowel series?

   a. To show the time of the day the exposure was made
   b. To indicate the interval between the exposure of the radiograph and the previous one
   c. To indicate the interval between the exposure of the radiograph and the ingestion of the barium

5. How should the patient be placed for timed radiographs when compression of the abdominal contents is desired?

   a. Prone
   b. Supine
   c. Lateral recumbent

6. Approximately how long after the patient swallows the barium sulfate mixture should the first radiograph be made?

   a. 5 minutes
   b. 15 minutes
   c. 30 minutes

7. Approximately how long after the exposure of the first radiograph should subsequent radiographs be exposed?

   a. 5 to 10 minutes
   b. 15 to 30 minutes
   c. 35 to 45 minutes

8. How might the oral method of small bowel examination be affected by giving the patient a cup of cold water after the administration of the contrast medium?

   a. Peristalsis is accelerated
   b. Peristalsis is slowed down
   c. The stomach becomes distended

9. Which small bowel series method often requires the administration of glucagon or diazepam (Valium) to relax the intestine and reduce patient discomfort during the initial filling of the small intestine?

   a. Oral
   b. Enteroclysis
   c. Complete reflux

10. How should the patient be positioned when the small intestine is to be filled by the complete reflux method?

    a. Prone
    b. Supine
    c. Lateral recumbent

11. Which small bowel series method injects contrast medium through an intestinal tube?

    a. Oral
    b. Enteroclysis
    c. Complete reflux

12. Where in the small intestine should the tube be inserted for the enteroclysis method of performing a small bowel series?

    a. Ileum
    b. Jejunum
    c. Duodenum

13. Which method of performing a small bowel series does not use a cleansing enema as part of patient preparation?

    a. Oral
    b. Enteroclysis
    c. Complete reflux

Items 14 through 20 pertain to the *AP or PA projection*. Examine Fig. 17-16 as you answer the following items.

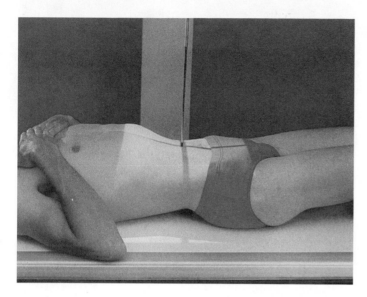

Figure 17-16 AP small intestine.

14. For the AP projection demonstrating the small intestine, which plane of the body should be centered to the grid?

   a. Horizontal
   b. Midsagittal
   c. Midcoronal

15. For the AP projection demonstrating the small intestine of a sthenic patient within 30 minutes after the administration of contrast, to which level of the patient should the IR be centered?

   a. T12
   b. L2
   c. L5

16. For delayed AP projections demonstrating the small intestine of a sthenic patient, to which level of the patient should the IR be centered?

   a. T12
   b. L2
   c. Iliac crests

17. For the AP projection, when should the exposure be made?

   a. At the end of expiration
   b. At the end of inspiration

18. How should the central ray be directed?

   a. Perpendicularly
   b. Angled caudally
   c. Angled cephalically

19. When visualized on a small bowel series radiograph, which structure usually indicates adequate demonstration of the entire small intestine?

   a. Cecum
   b. Jejunum
   c. Duodenum

20. From the following list, circle the seven evaluation criteria that indicate small bowel series radiographs were properly performed.

   a. The patient should not be rotated.
   b. A time marker should be included.
   c. No ribs should be seen below the diaphragm.
   d. The exposure factors should demonstrate the anatomy.
   e. The stomach should be included on the initial radiographs.
   f. The vertebral column should be in the middle of the radiograph.
   g. The entire small intestine should be included on each radiograph.
   h. The entire alimentary canal should be included on each radiograph.
   i. The examination is usually completed when barium is visualized in the cecum.
   j. The examination is usually completed when barium is visualized in the jejunum.
   k. The postevacuation film is accomplished after the administration of a cleansing enema.

Exercise 4: Large Intestine Examination

Instructions: The large intestine is frequently examined radiographically after the introduction of a suitable contrast medium. This type of examination is called the barium enema (BE). This exercise pertains to the procedures and radiographs used for the two methods of barium enemas. Identify structures, fill in missing words, provide a short answer, match columns, select from a list, or choose true or false (explaining any statement you believe to be false) for each item.

1. What are the two basic methods of performing a barium enema?

    a. Oral and double-contrast
    b. Oral and enteroclysis (intubation)
    c. Single-contrast and double-contrast
    d Single-contrast and enteroclysis (intubation)

2. What is the most common type of contrast medium used for a BE?

    BaSO4

3. Why should a high-density barium product be used as the contrast medium for double-contrast studies?

    Better coating of lumen

4. What two radiolucent contrast media can be used during the double-contrast study?

    Air & CO2

5. When might an orally administered, water-soluble, iodinated contrast medium be used in place of a barium sulfate mixture?

    —When pt. cannot tolerate retrograde filling

6. What should be included in the instructions generally given to a patient in preparation for a BE?

    — may vary
    — typical
    — Restrictive diet
    — laxatives
    — cleansing enema

7. What is considered the most important aspect of patient preparation for the BE?

    — Clean colon
    — no fecal material

8. What should the temperature of the barium be when the administration of a warm barium solution is desirable?

    85° - 90° F

9. How could the patient be affected if the barium solution is too warm?

    — irritating — may not be able to retain barium
    — may be injurious to tissue

10. What should the temperature of the barium be when administering cold barium solution?

41°F

11. What are the advantages of filling the large intestine with a cold barium solution?

- less irritation
- relaxes colon
- stimulate contraction of Anal sphincter

12. List three instructions that can be given to the patient to help the patient retain the barium during the examination.

- maintain contraction of Anal sphincter
- relax abdominal muscles
- concentrate on deep oral breathing

13. What is the maximum height above the level of the anus that a BE bag may be placed on a IV stand?

24" (61 cm)

14. Approximately how far into the rectum should an enema tip be inserted?

3½ - 4" (8.9 - 10 cm)

15. What wording refers to the last radiograph usually performed as part of a BE examination?

Post evac image

Items 16 through 19 pertain to the *PA projection.* Examine Fig. 17-17 as you answer the following items.

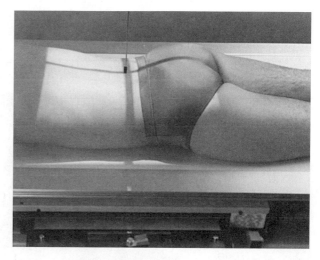

Figure 17-17 PA large intestine.

16. How should the patient be placed for the PA projection?
    a. Prone
    b. Supine
    c. Upright
    d. Lateral recumbent

17. To which level of the patient should the IR be centered?
    a. T12
    b. L2
    c. Iliac crests
    d. Symphysis pubis

18. How should the central ray be directed for the PA projection?
    a. Perpendicularly
    b. Angled caudally
    c. Angled cephalically

19. Identify each lettered structure shown in Fig. 17-18.

A. _____Left colic Flexure_____ (flexure)

B. _____Right " "_____ (flexure)

C. _____Transverse Colon_____

D. _____Descending "_____

E. _____Ascending "_____

F. _____Cecum_____

G. _____Sigmoid_____

H. _____Rectum_____

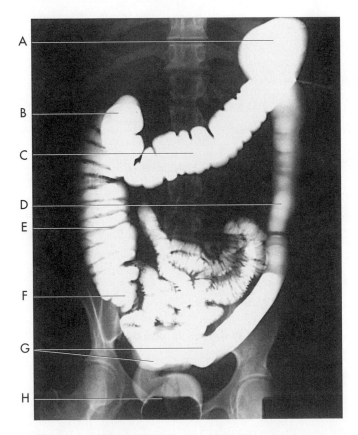

Figure 17-18 PA large intestine.

Items 20 through 25 pertain to the *PA axial projection.* Examine Fig. 17-19 as you answer the following items.

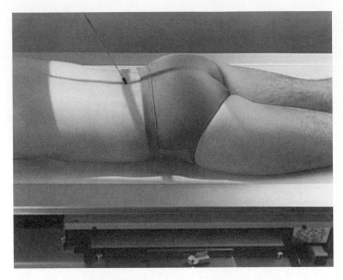

Figure 17-19 PA axial large intestine.

20. For the PA axial projection, which plane of the body should be centered to the midline of the table?

    a. Transverse
    b. Midsagittal
    c. Midcoronal

21. To which level of the patient should the central ray be directed for the PA axial projection?

    a. L2
    b. Symphysis pubis
    c. Anterior superior iliac spines

22. How should the central ray be directed for the PA axial projection?

    a. Perpendicularly
    b. Angled caudally
    c. Angled cephalically

23. Which area of the large intestine is best demonstrated with the PA axial projection?

    a. Ileocecal
    b. Superior
    c. Rectosigmoid

24. True or False. Both colic flexures should be seen with the PA axial projection.

25. Identify each lettered structure shown in Fig. 17-20.

   A. _____Splenic / Lt colic_____ (flexure)

   B. _____Transverse Colon_____

   C. _____Sigmoid_____

   D. _____Rectum_____

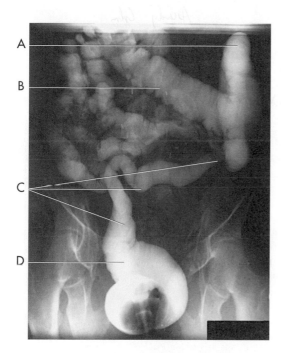

Figure 17-20 PA axial large intestine.

Items 26 through 30 pertain to the *PA oblique projection, RAO position.* Examine Fig. 17-21 as you answer the following items.

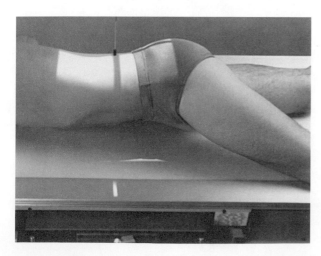

Figure 17-21 PA oblique large intestine, RAO position.

26. True or False. For the right PA oblique projection (RAO position), the patient should be rotated 35 to 45 degrees from the prone position.

27. True or False. For the right PA oblique projection (RAO position), the central ray should be directed 35 to 45 degrees caudally. 1

28. True or False. Both colic flexures should be seen in the RAO position radiograph.

29. True or False. The right PA oblique projection (RAO position) is performed primarily to demonstrate the right colic flexure.

30. Identify each lettered structure shown in Fig. 17-22.

   A. _____Splenic Flexure_____ (flexure)

   B. _____Hepatic Flexure_____ (flexure)

   C. _____Descending Colon_____

   D. _____Ascending Colon_____

   E. _____Sigmoid_____

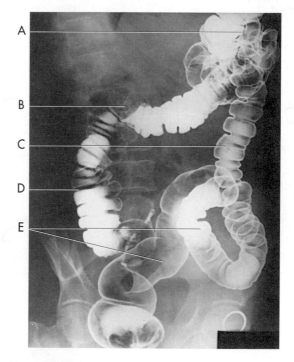

Figure 17-22 PA oblique large intestine, RAO position.

Items 31 through 33 pertain to the *PA oblique projection, LAO position*. Examine Fig. 17-23 as you answer the following items.

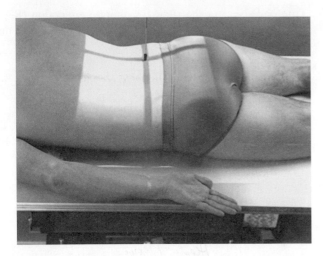

Figure 17-23 PA oblique large intestine, LAO position.

31. To which level of the patient should the IR be centered for the left PA oblique projection (LAO position)?

    a. T12
    b. L2
    c. Iliac crests
    d. Symphysis pubis

32. Which two structures of the large intestine are demonstrated primarily with the left PA oblique projection (LAO position)?

    a. Left colic flexure and ascending colon
    b. Left colic flexure and descending colon
    c. Right colic flexure and ascending colon
    d. Right colic flexure and descending colon

33. Identify each lettered structure shown in Fig. 17-24.

    A. _____Splenic Flexure_____ (flexure)

    B. _____Hepatic "_____ (flexure)

    C. _____Transverse Colon_____

    D. _____Descending Colon_____

    E. _____Ascending Colon_____

    F. _____Vermiform Appendix_____

    G. _____Sigmoid_____

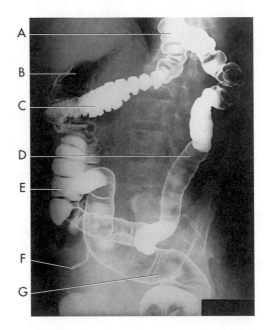

Figure 17-24 PA oblique large intestine, LAO position.

Items 34 through 38 pertain to the lateral projection. Examine Fig. 17-25 as you answer the following items.

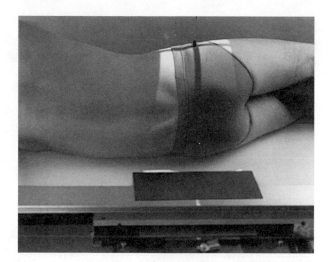

Figure 17-25 Left lateral rectum.

34. For the lateral projection, to what level of the patient should a IR that is 24 × 30 cm be centered?

level of ASIS

35. In the image of the left lateral projection, how is it determined that the patient was not rotated?

Hips / Femurs Are Superimposed

36. Which portions of the large intestine are of prime interest with the lateral projection?

a. Sigmoid and rectum
b. Cecum and ascending colon
c. Left colic flexure and descending colon
d. Right colic flexure and ascending colon

37. For the lateral projection, which plane of the body should be centered to the midline of the table?

a. Transverse
b. Midsagittal
c. Midcoronal

38. Identify each lettered structure shown in Fig. 17-26.

A. _Sigmoid_

B. _Sacrum_

C. _Rectum_

D. _Pubic Symphysis_

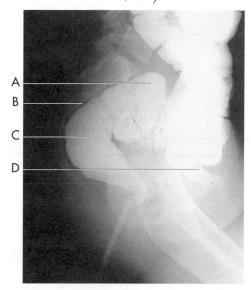

Figure 17-26 Left lateral rectum.

Items 39 through 43 pertain to the *AP projection*. Examine Fig. 17-27 as you answer the following items.

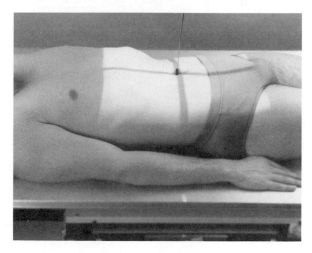

Figure 17-27 AP large intestine.

39. Which plane of the body should be centered to the grid for the AP projection?

Mid sagittal

40. To what level of the patient should the IR be centered?

iliac Crests

41. True or False. The patient should suspend respiration for the exposure.

42. True or False. The entire colon should be demonstrated for the AP projection.

43. Identify each lettered structure shown in Fig. 17-28.

A. _____ Splenic Flexure _____ (flexure)

B. _____ transverse Colon _____

C. _____ Hepatic Plexure _____ (flexure)

D. _____ Descending Colon _____

E. _____ Ascending colon _____

F. _____ Sigmoid _____

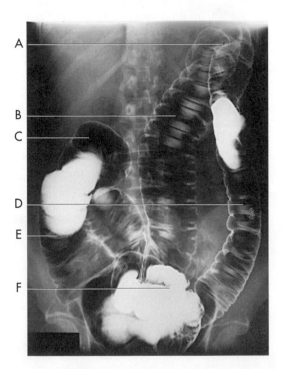

Figure 17-28 AP large intestine.

Items 44 through 48 pertain to the *AP axial projection*. Examine Fig. 17-29 as you answer the following items.

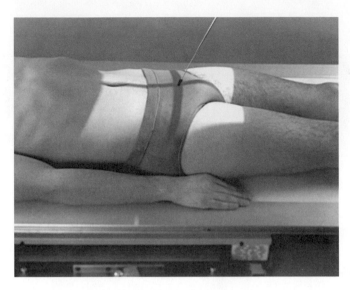

Figure 17-29 AP axial large intestine.

44. Which projection produces an image similar to the AP axial projection?

a. AP projection
b. PA axial projection
c. Left PA oblique projection, LAO position
d. Right PA oblique projection, RAO position

45. In which direction and how many degrees should the central ray be directed?

a. Caudally 10 to 20 degrees
b. Caudally 30 to 40 degrees
c. Cephalically 10 to 20 degrees
d. Cephalically 30 to 40 degrees

46. For the AP axial projection, where on the patient's anterior surface should the central ray enter when a 35 × 43 cm IR is used?

    2" ↓ ASIS

47. To produce a coned-down image of the AP axial projection on an image receptor that is 24 × 30 cm, where on the patient should the central ray enter?

    - inferior margin of public symphysis

48. Identify each lettered structure shown in Fig. 17-30.

    A. _____Descending colon_____

    B. _____Sigmoid_____

    C. _____Rectum_____

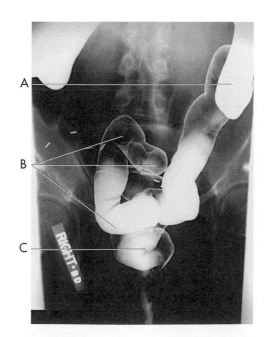

Figure 17-30 AP axial large intestine.

Items 49 through 53 pertain to the *AP oblique projection, LPO position.* Examine Fig. 17-31 as you answer the following items.

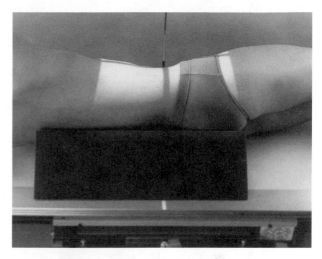

Figure 17-31 AP oblique large intestine, LPO position.

49. The left AP oblique projection (LPO position) produces an image similar to the _____RAO_____ PA oblique projection (_____RAO_____ position).

50. For the left AP oblique projection (LPO position), the patient should be rotated _35_ to _45_ degrees.

51. For the left AP oblique projection (LPO position), which side of the patient—right or left—should be elevated away from the x-ray table?

    Right

52. Which flexure—right colic or left colic—should be well demonstrated with the left AP oblique projection (LPO position)?

    Right colic

53. Identify each lettered structure shown in Fig. 17-32.

A. _____Splenic Flexure_____ (flexure)

B. _____Hepatic Flexure._____ (flexure)

C. _____Descending Colon_____

D. _____Ascending Colon_____

E. _____Sigmoid_____

F. _____Rectum_____

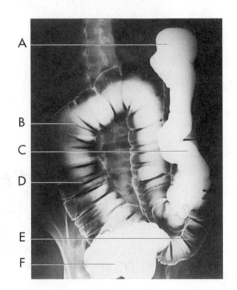

Figure 17-32 AP oblique large intestine, LPO position.

Items 54 through 57 pertain to the *AP oblique projection (right posterior oblique [RPO] position)*. Examine Fig. 17-33 as you answer the following items.

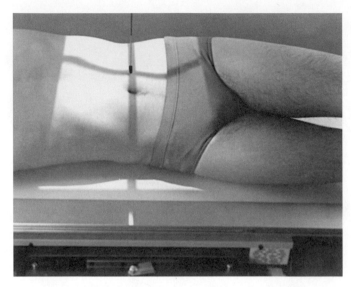

Figure 17-33 AP oblique large intestine, RPO position.

54. What other oblique position produces an image similar to the right AP oblique projection (RPO position)?

LAO

55. Which flexure—right colic or left colic—should be well demonstrated with the right AP oblique projection (RPO position)?

Lt - Colic

56. How many degrees should the patient be rotated from the supine position for the right AP oblique projection (RPO position)?

35 - 45°

57. Identify each lettered structure shown in Fig. 17-34.

A. _____ *Splenic* _____ (flexure)

B. _____ *Transverse* _____

C. _____ *Hepatic* _____ (flexure)

D. _____ *Descending colon* _____

E. _____ *Ascending colon* _____

F. _____ *Sigmoid* _____

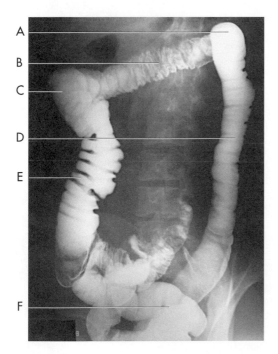

Figure 17-34 AP oblique large intestine, RPO position.

Items 58 through 64 pertain to *AP or PA projections, right and left lateral decubitus positions.* Examine Figs. 17-35 and 17-36 as you answer the following items.

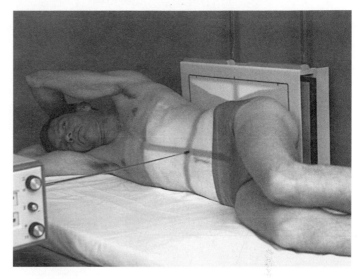

Figure 17-35 AP large intestine, right lateral decubitus position.

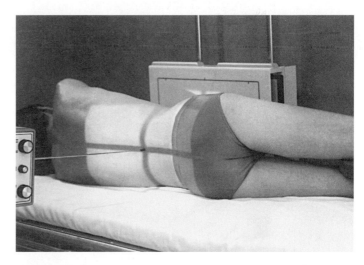

Figure 17-36 PA large intestine, left lateral decubitus position.

58. Which BE projection requires that the patient be placed in the right lateral recumbent position and that a horizontal central ray be directed to the midline of the patient at the level of the iliac crests?
   a. Right lateral
   b. Right AP oblique (RPO position)
   c. Right PA oblique (RAO position)
   d. AP, right lateral decubitus position

59. For lateral decubitus positions, what should be accomplished to ensure that the dependent side of the patient is demonstrated?

Support pt. on A Radiolucent pad

60. How much of the colon should be demonstrated in the image of a lateral decubitus position?

Area from flexure to rectum

61. Name the lateral decubitus position that best demonstrates each of the following intestinal structures.

a. Left colic flexure: _Rt Lat Decub_

b. Right colic flexure: _Lt - Lat Decub_

62. Figs. 17-37 and 17-38 are lateral decubitus radiographs. Examine the images and answer the questions that follow.

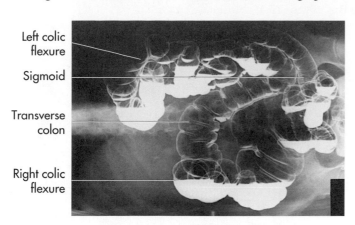

Left colic flexure
Sigmoid
Transverse colon
Right colic flexure

Figure 17-37 Radiograph of the large intestine, lateral decubitus position.

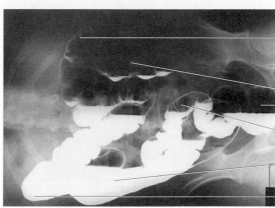

Right colic flexure
Ascending colon
Rectum
Sigmoid
Descending colon
Left colic flexure

Figure 17-38 Radiograph of the large intestine, lateral decubitus position.

a. Which image shows the left lateral decubitus position?

_____ 17-38 _____

b. Which image shows the right lateral decubitus position?

_____ 17-37 _____

c. Which image best demonstrates the left colic flexure?

_____ 17-37 _____

d. Which image best demonstrates the right colic flexure?

_____ 17-38 _____

e. Which image requires that the patient be placed in the left lateral recumbent position?

_____ 17-38 _____

f. Which image requires that the patient be placed in the right lateral recumbent position?

_____ 17-37 _____

Questions 63 and 64 pertain to BE radiographs performed with the patient in the upright position.

63. For upright frontal, oblique, and lateral projections, how is the centering of the IR adjusted from that used for the recumbent positions? Why is this compensation necessary?

lower due to gravity

64. Examine Fig. 17-39 and answer the questions that follow.

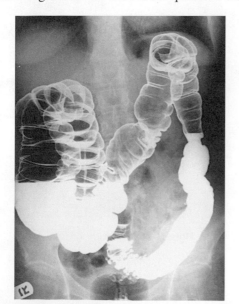

Figure 17-39 AP large intestine.

a. What body position was used to make this radiograph?

upright

b. What image characteristics led you to that conclusion?

– Barium seen settling to lower levels of colon

65. Figs. 17-40 through 17-47 represent different projections used to obtain BE radiographs. Examine the images, then match the figures in Column A with the positions/projections in Column B.

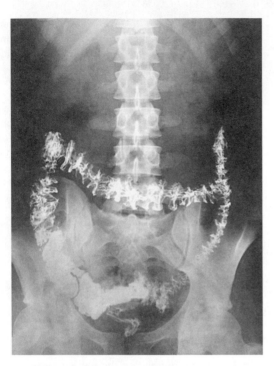

Figure 17-40 BE radiograph.

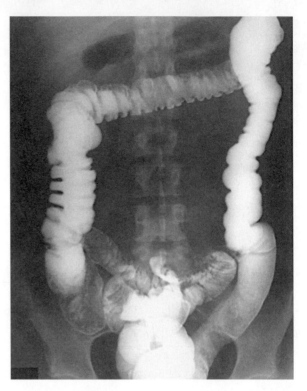

Figure 17-42 BE radiograph.

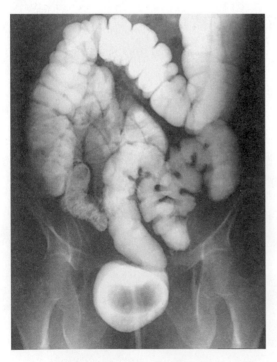

Figure 17-41 BE radiograph.

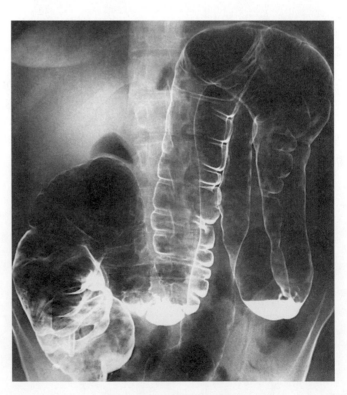

Figure 17-43 BE radiograph.

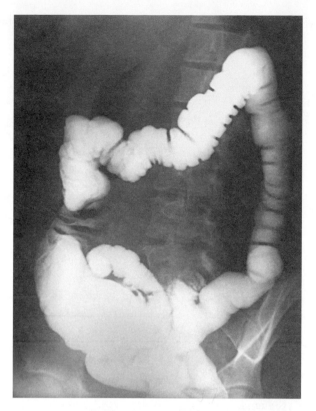

Figure 17-44 BE radiograph.

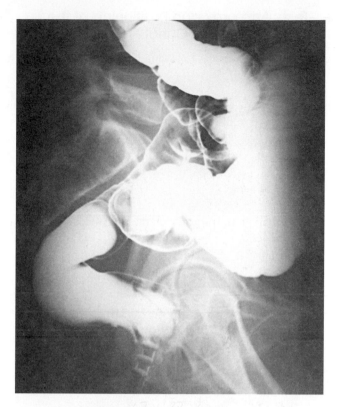

Figure 17-46 BE radiograph.

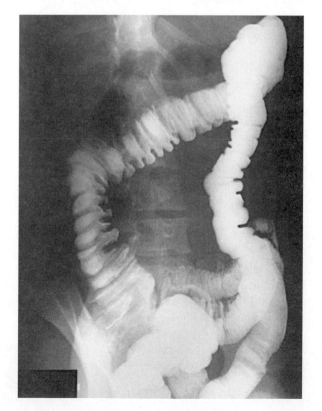

Figure 17-45 BE radiograph.

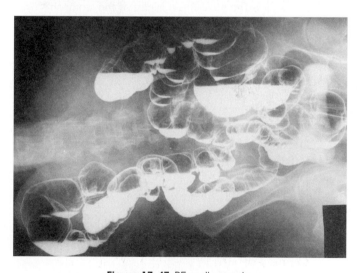

Figure 17-47 BE radiograph.

Column A	Column B
_G_ 1. Fig. 17-40	a. LAO position
_C_ 2. Fig. 17-41	b. LPO position
_E_ 3. Fig. 17-42	c. AP, axial projection
_D_ 4. Fig. 17-43	d. PA, upright position
_A_ 5. Fig. 17-44	e. AP, recumbent position
_B_ 6. Fig. 17-45	f. Left lateral position
_F_ 7. Fig. 17-46	g. Postevacuation
_H_ 8. Fig. 17-47	h. Lateral decubitus position

Self-Test: Anatomy and Positioning of the Alimentary Canal

Instructions: Answer the following questions by selecting the best choice.

1. In which body habitus type is the stomach almost horizontal and high in the abdomen?

   a. Sthenic
   b. Asthenic
   c. Hyposthenic
   d. Hypersthenic

2. Which curvature is located on the right (medial) border of the stomach?

   a. Lesser
   b. Greater
   c. Inferior
   d. Superior

3. Which area is the most superior part of the stomach?

   a. Head
   b. Body
   c. Fundus
   d. Pylorus

4. Which area is the most inferior part of the stomach?

   a. Body
   b. Cardia
   c. Fundus
   d. Pylorus

5. The distal esophagus empties its contents into which of the following?

   a. Duodenum
   b. Pyloric canal
   c. Duodenal bulb
   d. Cardiac antrum

6. Which opening is located between the stomach and small intestine?

   a. Cardiac orifice
   b. Pyloric orifice
   c. Ileocecal orifice
   d. Ampulla of Vater

7. Which opening is at the distal end of the small intestine?

   a. Anus
   b. Cardiac orifice
   c. Pyloric orifice
   d. Ileocecal orifice

8. Which structure is the proximal part of the small intestine?

   a. Ileum
   b. Pylorus
   c. Jejunum
   d. Duodenum

9. Which structure is the distal part of the small intestine?

   a. Ileum
   b. Cecum
   c. Jejunum
   d. Duodenum

10. In which abdominal region does the large intestine originate?

    a. Left iliac
    b. Right iliac
    c. Left lumbar
    d. Right lumbar

11. Which structure is the proximal part of the large intestine?

    a. Ileum
    b. Cecum
    c. Rectum
    d. Sigmoid

12. Which part of the large intestine is located between the ascending and descending parts of the colon?

    a. Cecum
    b. Rectum
    c. Sigmoid
    d. Transverse colon

13. Which structure is located between the ascending colon and the transverse colon?

    a. Sigmoid
    b. Left colic flexure
    c. Right colic flexure
    d. Descending colon

14. Where in the large intestine is the left colic flexure located?

    a. Between the cecum and the ascending colon
    b. Between the ascending colon and the transverse colon
    c. Between the transverse colon and the descending colon
    d. Between the descending colon and the sigmoid

15. Which structure is the pouchlike part of the large intestine situated below the junction of the ileum and the colon?

    a. Cecum
    b. Rectum
    c. Sigmoid
    d. Veriform appendix

16. Where in the large intestine is the sigmoid located?

    a. Between the cecum and the transverse colon
    b. Between the ascending colon and the transverse colon
    c. Between the descending colon and the rectum
    d. Between the transverse colon and the descending colon

17. Approximately how long does it usually take a barium meal to reach the ileocecal valve?

    a. 30 minutes to 1 hour
    b. 2 to 3 hours
    c. 4 to 5 hours
    d. 24 hours

18. Approximately how long does it usually take a barium meal to reach the rectum?

    a. 2 to 3 hours
    b. 4 to 5 hours
    c. 6 to 8 hours
    d. 24 hours

19. Which two imaging modalities are most commonly used to examine the alimentary canal after the introduction of a barium product?

    a. Fluoroscopy and sonography
    b. Fluoroscopy and radiography
    c. Computed tomography and sonography
    d. Computed tomography and radiography

20. Which type of contrast medium is most commonly used for examining the upper GI tract?

    a. An oily, viscous compound
    b. A barium sulfate suspension
    c. A nonionic injectable compound
    d. A water-soluble, iodinated solution

21. To best demonstrate the swallowing function, in which position should the patient be placed to begin the fluoroscopic phase of single-contrast examinations of the esophagus?

    a. Upright
    b. Left lateral decubitus
    c. Recumbent LAO
    d. Recumbent RPO

22. Which two recumbent oblique positions can be used to best demonstrate an unobstructed image of a barium-filled esophagus between the vertebrae and the heart?

    a. LAO and LPO
    b. LAO and RPO
    c. RAO and LPO
    d. RAO and RPO

23. Which of the following is a major advantage of the double-contrast UGI examination over the single-contrast UGI examination?

    a. The patient can better tolerate the procedure.
    b. Radiation exposure to the patient is reduced.
    c. Small lesions on the mucosal lining are better demonstrated.
    d. The examination can be performed with the patient upright instead of recumbent

24. Which description refers to the biphasic GI examination?

    a. A single-contrast study of the entire alimentary canal
    b. A single-contrast study of the upper GI tract
    c. A double-contrast study of the upper GI tract
    d. A combination single-contrast and double-contrast study of the upper GI tract

25. Which body habitus produces the greatest visceral movement when a patient is moved from the prone position to the upright position?

    a. Sthenic
    b. Asthenic
    c. Hyposthenic
    d. Hypersthenic

26. For the PA projection as part of the UGI examination, why should the lower lung fields be included on a 35 × 43 cm image receptor?

    a. To demonstrate pneumothorax
    b. To demonstrate a possible hiatal hernia
    c. To demonstrate fluid levels in the thorax
    d. To demonstrate the gas bubble in the fundus of the stomach

27. For the double-contrast UGI examination, which projection produces the best image of a gas-filled duodenal bulb and pyloric canal?

    a. Left AP oblique projection (LPO position) with the patient upright
    b. Left AP oblique projection (LPO position) with the patient recumbent
    c. Right PA oblique projection (RAO position) with the patient upright
    d. Right PA oblique projection (RAO position) with the patient recumbent

28. For the single-contrast UGI examination with the patient recumbent, which projection produces the best image of a barium-filled pyloric canal and duodenal bulb in patients whose habitus approximates the sthenic type?

    a. AP projection
    b. Left lateral projection
    c. Left AP oblique projection (LPO position)
    d. Right PA oblique projection (RAO position)

29. For the UGI examination with the patient recumbent, which projection best stimulates gastric peristalsis to better demonstrate the pyloric canal and duodenal bulb?

    a. AP projection
    b. Left lateral projection
    c. Left AP oblique projection (LPO position)
    d. Right PA oblique projection (RAO position)

30. Which breathing procedure should the patient perform when UGI radiographs are exposed?

    a. Slow, deep breathing
    b. Quick, panting breaths
    c. Suspended expiration
    d. Suspended inspiration

31. For the double-contrast UGI examination with the patient recumbent, which projection produces the best image of a gas-filled fundus?

    a. Left lateral projection
    b. AP projection, left lateral decubitus position
    c. Left AP oblique projection (LPO position)
    d. Right PA oblique projection (RAO position)

32. For the UGI examination with the patient recumbent, which projection best demonstrates the right retrogastric space?

    a. Right lateral projection
    b. AP projection, right lateral decubitus position
    c. Left AP oblique projection (LPO position)
    d. Right PA oblique projection (RAO position)

33. For the AP projection with the patient supine (as part of the UGI examination), which procedure should be performed to best demonstrate a diaphragmatic herniation (hiatal hernia)?

    a. Angle the central ray 30 to 35 degrees caudally.
    b. Tilt the table and patient into a full Trendelenburg position.
    c. Instruct the patient to suspend respiration after full inspiration.
    d. Place radiolucent cushions under the thorax to elevate the shoulders.

34. To which level of the patient should the central ray be directed for the right PA oblique projection (RAO position) as part of the UGI examination?

    a. T9–T10
    b. T11–T12
    c. L1–L2
    d. L3–L4

35. Which examination of the alimentary canal requires that a series of radiographs be taken at specific time intervals after the ingestion of the contrast medium?

    a. UGI series
    b. Barium enema
    c. Esophagography
    d. Small bowel series

36. For a small bowel series of a patient with hypomotility of the small intestine, which procedure should be performed to accelerate peristalsis?

    a. Roll the patient 360 degrees.
    b. Instruct the patient to drink a glass of ice water.
    c. Instruct the patient to perform the Valsalva maneuver.
    d. Tilt the table and patient into a full Trendelenburg position.

37. Which structure, when visualized on a radiograph as part of a small bowel series, usually indicates the completion of the exam?

    a. Ileum
    b. Cecum
    c. Jejunum
    d. Duodenum

38. What is the proper sequence for filling the large intestine with barium when performing a BE?

    a. Rectum, sigmoid, ascending colon, transverse colon, and descending colon
    b. Rectum, sigmoid, descending colon, transverse colon, and ascending colon
    c. Sigmoid, rectum, ascending colon, transverse colon, and descending colon
    d. Sigmoid, rectum, descending colon, transverse colon, and ascending colon

39. Which procedure should be used during a BE to relax the large intestine and enable the patient to better retain the barium sulfate suspension?

    a. Instruct the patient to perform the Valsalva maneuver.
    b. Raise the barium bag to 24 inches above the rectum.
    c. Administer cold (41°F) barium sulfate suspension.
    d. Administer warm (95°F) barium sulfate suspension.

40. Before the enema tip is inserted during a BE, why should a small amount of barium sulfate mixture be allowed to run into a waste basin?

    a. To lubricate the enema tip
    b. To remove air from the tube
    c. To determine if the mixture is too warm or too cold
    d. To ensure that the consistency of the mixture is adequate

41. Which procedure should be accomplished when inserting the enema tip for a BE?

    a. Lubricate the tip with petroleum jelly.
    b. Place the patient in the Trendelenburg position.
    c. Inflate the air-filled retention tip before insertion.
    d. Ensure that the tip is inserted no more than $3\frac{1}{2}$ to 4 inches (8.9 to 10 cm).

42. For the PA projection during a BE, what is the advantage of placing the x-ray table and patient in a slight Trendelenburg position?

    a. To demonstrate the ileocecal valve
    b. To enable more air to be injected into the colon
    c. To help separate overlapping loops of distal bowel
    d. To move the transverse colon higher in the abdomen

43. Which structures of the large intestine are of primary interest with AP axial or PA axial projections during a BE?

    a. Sigmoid and rectum
    b. Cecum and ileocecal valve
    c. Left and right colic flexures
    d. Ascending and descending colons

44. How many degrees and in which direction should the central ray be directed for the PA axial projection during a BE?

    a. 20 to 25 degrees caudal
    b. 20 to 25 degrees cephalic
    c. 30 to 40 degrees caudal
    d. 30 to 40 degrees cephalic

45. Which structure of the large intestine is of primary interest for the right PA oblique projection (RAO position) during BE examinations?

    a. Anal canal
    b. Left colic flexure
    c. Right colic flexure
    d. Descending colon

46. Which two oblique projections can be performed to best demonstrate the left colic flexure during a BE?

    a. Left PA oblique projection (LAO position) and left AP oblique projection (LPO position)
    b. Left PA oblique projection (LAO position) and right AP oblique projection (RPO position)
    c. Right PA oblique projection (RAO position) and left AP oblique projection (LPO position)
    d. Right PA oblique projection (RAO position) and right AP oblique projection (RPO position)

47. Which structure of the large intestine is best demonstrated if the patient is rotated 45 degrees from a supine position to move the right side of the abdomen away from the x-ray table during a BE?

    a. Ileum
    b. Cecum
    c. Left colic flexure
    d. Right colic flexure

48. For the right lateral decubitus position as part of a barium enema, which procedure should be done to ensure that the ascending colon is demonstrated in the image?

    a. Center the IR to the iliac crests.
    b. Elevate the patient on a radiolucent support.
    c. Tilt the table and patient into a full Trendelenburg position.
    d. Make the exposure after the patient suspends respiration.

49. Which BE projection requires that a 24 × 30 cm IR be placed lengthwise and centered to the level of the anterior-superior iliac spine (ASIS)?

    a. AP projection
    b. Lateral projection
    c. AP projection, left lateral decubitus position
    d. Left AP oblique projection (LPO position)

50. Which BE projection does not require colic flexures to be included in the image?

    a. AP projection
    b. Lateral projection
    c. AP projection, lateral decubitus position
    d Right PA oblique projection (RAO position)

CHAPTER 18

Urinary System

SECTION 1

Anatomy of the Urinary System

Exercise 1

Instructions: This exercise pertains to urinary structures. Identify structures for each question.

1. Identify each lettered structure shown in Fig. 18-1.

   A. _____

   B. _____

   C. _____

   D. _____

   E. _____

   F. _____

2. Identify each lettered structure shown in Fig. 18-2.

   A. _____

   B. _____

   C. _____

   D. _____

   E. _____

   F. _____

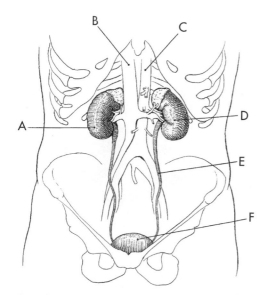

Figure 18-1 Anterior aspect of the urinary system in relation to the surrounding structures.

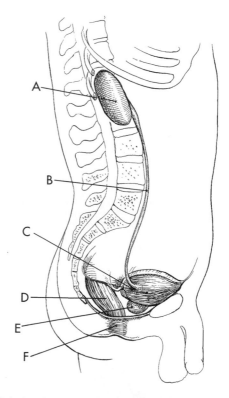

Figure 18-2 Lateral aspect of the male urinary system in relation to the surrounding structures.

3. Identify each lettered part of the kidney shown in Fig. 18-3.

A. _____   F. _____

B. _____   G. _____

C. _____   H. _____

D. _____   I. _____

E. _____

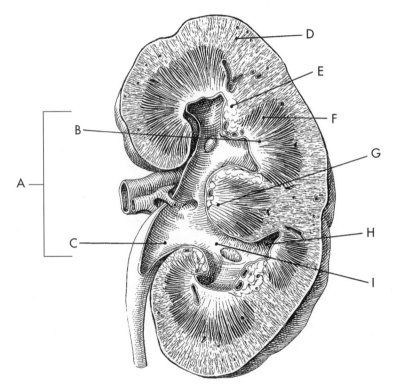

Figure 18-3 Midcoronal section of a kidney.

4. Identify each lettered structure shown in Fig. 18-4.

A. _____

B. _____

C. _____

D. _____

E. _____

F. _____

G. _____

H. _____

I. _____

J. _____

K. _____

5. Identify each lettered structure shown in Fig. 18-5.

A. _____

B. _____

C. _____

D. _____

E. _____

F. _____

G. _____

H. _____

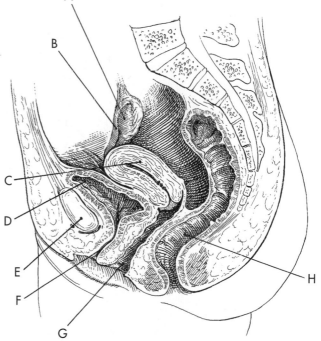

Figure 18-5 Midsagittal section through the female pelvis.

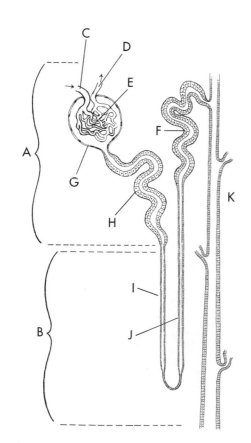

Figure 18-4 Diagram of a nephron and collecting duct.

6. Identify each lettered structure shown in Fig. 18-6.

A. _____   D. _____

B. _____   E. _____

C. _____   F. _____

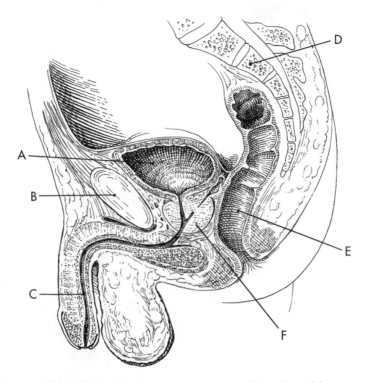

Figure 18-6 Midsagittal section through the male pelvis.

Exercise 2

Instructions: Use the following clues to complete the crossword puzzle. All answers refer to the urinary system.

ACROSS

3. Outer renal tissue
4. This arteriole leaves the capsule
6. Filtrate derivative
7. Another term for suprarenal
8. Urine vessel from glomerular capsule
10. Cup-shaped urine receivers
12. Cone-shaped renal segments
15. Cluster of blood vessels
16. Urinary reservoir
17. Functional renal unit
18. Musculomembranous excretory duct
19. Medial opening of a kidney

DOWN

1. This arteriole enters the capsule
2. Inner renal tissue
3. Membranous cup; Bowman's _____
5. Central renal cavity
6. External excretory tube
9. Male gland
11. Gland that is found on a kidney
13. Glomerular fluid
14. Primary organ of urinary system

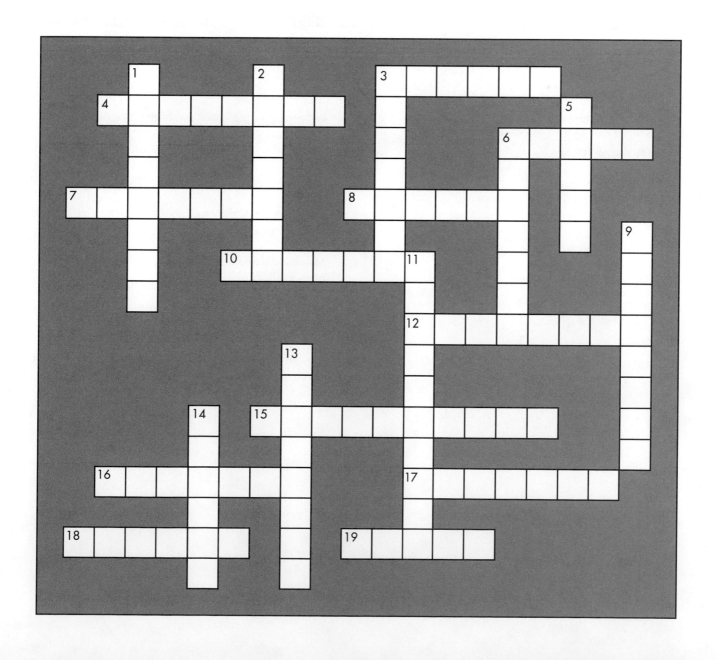

Exercise 3

Instructions: Match the pathology terms in Column A with the appropriate definition in Column B. Not all choices from Column B should be selected.

Column A

_____ 1. Tumor

_____ 2. Fistula

_____ 3. Cystitis

_____ 4. Stenosis

_____ 5. Calculus

_____ 6. Carcinoma

_____ 7. Ureterocele

_____ 8. Pyelonephritis

_____ 9. Hydronephrosis

_____ 10. Polycystic kidney

_____ 11. Renal obstruction

_____ 12. Renal hypertension

_____ 13. Glomerulonephritis

_____ 14. Congenital anomaly

_____ 15. Vesicoureteral reflux

Column B

a. Inflammation of the bladder

b. Enlargement of the prostrate

c. Abnormality present since birth

d. Narrowing or contraction of a passage

e. Increased blood pressure to the kidneys

f. Inflammation of the kidney and renal pelvis

g. Malignant new growth composed of epithelial cells

h. Distension of the renal pelvis and calyces with urine

i. Backward flow of urine from the bladder into the ureters

j. Ballooning of the lower end of the ureter into the bladder

k. Abnormal concretion of mineral salts, often called a stone

l. New tissue growth where cell proliferation is uncontrolled

m. Inflammation of the capillary loops in the glomeruli of the kidneys

n. Massive enlargement of the kidney with the formation of many cysts

o. Condition preventing the normal flow of urine through the urinary system

p. Abnormal connection between two internal organs or between an organ and the body surface

Exercise 4

Instructions: This exercise pertains to the anatomy of the urinary system. Fill in missing words for each question.

1. The kidneys and ureters are part of the

   _____ system.

2. The organ that removes waste products from the blood is

   the _____.

3. The gland that sits on the superior pole of each kidney is

   the _____ gland.

4. Blood vessels, nerves, and the ureter enter a kidney

   through an opening known as the _____.

5. The hilum is located on the _____ border
   of the kidney.

6. In the average (sthenic) person, the superior pole of the

   kidney is located at the _____ vertebral
   level.

7. The microscopic functional unit of the kidney is the

   _____.

8. Nephron units are found in the layer of renal tissue known

   as the _____.

9. The proximal portion of a nephron consisting of a double-

   walled membranous cup is the _____
   capsule.

10. A cluster of blood capillaries surrounded by a Bowman's

    capsule is a _____.

11. A glomerulus branches off the _____
    artery.

12. The blood vessel entering a glomerular capsule is the

    _____ arteriole; the blood vessel leav-

    ing a glomerular capsule is the _____
    arteriole.

13. The fluid that passes from the glomerulus to the glomeru-

    lar capsule is _____

    _____.

14. Urine from collecting ducts drains into minor

    _____.

15. Minor calyces drain urine into major _____.

16. Major calyces unite to form the expanded, funnel-shaped

    renal _____.

17. The long tubes that transport urine from the kidneys are the

    _____.

18. Ureters transport urine from kidneys to the

    _____ _____.

19. The musculomembranous tube that conveys urine from
    the urinary bladder to outside the body is the

    _____.

20. The gland that surrounds the proximal part of the male ure-

    thra is the _____.

Exercise 5: Venipuncture and IV Contrast Media Administration

Instructions: This exercise pertains to venipuncture and intravenous (IV) contrast media administration. Items require you to write a short answer or select from a list.

1. Which condition should be prevented if strict aseptic techniques are used when administering medications intravenously?

   a. The patient lapsing into shock
   b. Introducing infection into the patient
   c. Injecting an excessive amount of medication

2. How does the use of an IV filter affect a bolus injection?

   a. The rate of injection will be reduced.
   b. The introduction of foreign matter will increase.
   c. The time required to inject the medication will be reduced.

3. What are the three parts of a syringe?

   a. Tip, barrel, and bevel
   b. Tip, barrel, and plunger
   c. Hub, cannula, and bevel
   d. Hub, cannula, and plunger

4. What are the three parts of a hypodermic needle?

   a. Tip, barrel, and bevel
   b. Tip, barrel, and plunger
   c. Hub, cannula, and bevel
   d. Hub, cannula, and plunger

5. What does the term *needle gauge* refer to?

   a. The angle of the bevel
   b. The length of the needle
   c. The diameter of the needle

6. What injection apparatus is preferred for most IV administrations?

   a. Butterfly set
   b. Over-the-needle cannula
   c. Seldinger-technique needle

7. Which procedure should be performed to maintain a closed system with a multiple-dose vial of medication?

   a. Discard the vial after the second use.
   b. Inject into the bottle an amount of air equal to the amount of fluid to be withdrawn.
   c. Inject into the bottle an amount of sterile saline solution equal to the amount of fluid to be withdrawn.

8. When assessing vessels for venipuncture, why should a vessel not be used if a pulse is detected?

   a. A pulse indicates the vessel is an artery.
   b. A pulse indicates the patient is hypertensive.
   c. A pulse indicates the patient has low blood pressure.
   d. A pulse indicates the patient has a fistula in that vessel.

9. From the following list, circle the four sites that are most often used for establishing IV access.

   a. Anterior hand
   b. Posterior hand
   c. Femoral artery
   d. Anterior forearm
   e. Posterior forearm
   f. Ulnar aspect of the wrist
   g. Radial aspect of the wrist
   h. Anterior aspect of the elbow

10. Describe how the skin should be prepared before inserting a needle into a vein.

11. How far above the site of a venipuncture should the tourniquet be placed?

12. How should the IV needle be inserted—bevel up or bevel down?

13. When inserting an IV needle into the patient, what angle should exist between the needle and the patient's skin surface?

14. What is the significance of a backflow of blood into the syringe during a venipuncture procedure?

15. What procedure should a radiographer perform if the needle has punctured both walls of the vein?

16. What is infiltration?

    a. The procedure for using an IV filter in tubing
    b. The introduction of a hypodermic needle into a vein
    c. The process of injecting fluid into tissues instead of a vein

17. Which other term refers to infiltration?

    a. Extraction
    b. Extirpation
    c. Extravasation

18. Which procedure should a radiographer perform after a needle has been removed from a vein?

    a. Apply a tourniquet 3 to 4 inches above the puncture site.
    b. Using a 2 × 2 pad of gauze, apply pressure directly to the injection site.
    c. Clean the area using a circular motion covering an area that is approximately 2 inches in diameter.

19. From the following list, circle the four symptoms that may indicate the occurrence of infiltration.

    a. Pain
    b. Burning
    c. Redness
    d. Swelling
    e. Dyspnea
    f. Sneezing
    g. Rapid pulse
    h. Hypotension

20. From the following list, circle the five golden rules of medication administration.

    a. The right time
    b. The right route
    c. The right patient
    d. The right syringe
    e. The right amount
    f. The right medication
    g. The right technologist
    h. The right body position

SECTION 2

Positioning of the Urinary System

Exercise 1: Excretory Urography

Instructions: Radiography of the urinary system comprises numerous specialized procedures. The most common radiographic examination of the urinary system is the excretory urogram. This exercise pertains to excretory urography. Identify structures, fill in missing words, select from a list, provide a short answer, or choose true or false (explain any item you believe to be false) for each question.

Questions 1 through 22 pertain to general information concerning excretory urography.

1. The radiographic investigation of the renal drainage system is accomplished by various procedures classified under the general term of _____.

2. Which two terms refer to the excretory urogram examination?

   a. Cystourethrography and retrograde urography
   b. Cystourethrography and intravenous pyelography
   c. Intravenous urography and retrograde urography
   d. Intravenous urography and intravenous pyelography

3. From the following list, circle four terms that identify the typical contrast media currently used in excretory urography.

   a. Ionic
   b. Nonionic
   c. Iodinated
   d. Noniodinated
   e. Injectable
   f. Noninjectable

4. From the following list, circle the mild adverse reactions to iodinated contrast medium administration.

   a. Hives
   b. Death
   c. Nausea
   d. Dyspnea
   e. Vomiting
   f. Warm feeling
   g. Cardiac arrest
   h. Renal shutdown
   i. Respiratory arrest
   j. Flushed appearance
   k. Edema of the respiratory mucous membranes

5. How soon after the injection of a contrast medium are symptoms of a reaction most likely to occur?

   a. Within 5 minutes
   b. Between 5 to 10 minutes
   c. More than 10 minutes

6. From the following list, circle the four typical procedures that a patient might ideally experience when preparing for the intravenous urography (IVU) examination.

   a. Laxative
   b. Cleansing enema
   c. Light evening meal
   d. Liquid diet for 3 to 4 days
   e. Low-residue diet for 1 or 2 days
   f. Drinking 32 ounces of water to fill the bladder
   g. Nothing by mouth (NPO) after midnight on the day of the examination

7. What is the purpose of giving a child 12 ounces of carbonated beverage just before the start of IVU?

8. Why should an immobilization band not be applied across the patient's upper abdomen in an effort to control motion during IVU?

9. What is the purpose of applying compression over the distal ends of the ureters?

10. Where on the abdomen should compression pads be located to compress the ureters?

11. When ureteral compression is used, why should the pressure be slowly released when the compression device is no longer needed?

12. Why is ureteral compression currently not often used in excretory urography?

13. Why might an upright anteroposterior (AP) projection of the abdomen be made *before* the injection of the contrast medium?

14. What identification data should be included on every postinjection radiograph?

15. Why is it desirable to have the patient remove his or her underwear?

16. Why should the patient be instructed to empty his or her bladder just before IVU is to begin?

    a. To locate the ureteral openings
    b. To measure the capacity of the bladder
    c. To prevent dilution of the opacified urine

17. From the following list, circle the five reasons that AP projections with the patient recumbent are performed as the scout radiograph.

    a. To demonstrate the bladder
    b. To identify the location of the kidneys
    c. To demonstrate the presence of calculi
    d. To demonstrate the contour of the kidneys
    e. To check the radiographic exposure factors
    f. To demonstrate the mobility of the kidneys
    g. To examine for radiopaque artifacts on the positioning table
    h. To determine how well the patient's gastrointestinal (GI) tract was cleaned

18. What can be done to enhance the filling of renal structures with contrast medium when the patient is supine?

    a. Place supports under the patient's knees.
    b. Place a support under the patient's lumbar region.
    c. Direct the central ray 20 to 25 degrees caudally.
    d. Tilt the x-ray table and patient to the Trendelenburg position.

19. Approximately how long after a bolus injection of the contrast medium should the exposure be made to best demonstrate a nephrogram?

    a. 30 seconds
    b. 3 minutes
    c. 5 minutes

20. How long after the completion of the contrast medium injection does the contrast agent usually begin to appear in the renal pelvis?

    a. 30 seconds to 1 minute
    b. 2 to 8 minutes
    c. 10 to 14 minutes
    d. 15 to 20 minutes

21. How long after the injection of the contrast medium does the greatest concentration usually appear within the kidneys?

    a. 30 seconds to 1 minute
    b. 2 to 8 minutes
    c. 15 to 20 minutes
    d. 30 to 45 minutes

22. A postvoiding radiograph is usually the last radiograph taken to demonstrate which structure(s)?

    a. Ureters
    b. Bladder
    c. Kidneys

Items 23 through 32 pertain to the *AP projection.* Examine Fig. 18-7 as you answer the following items.

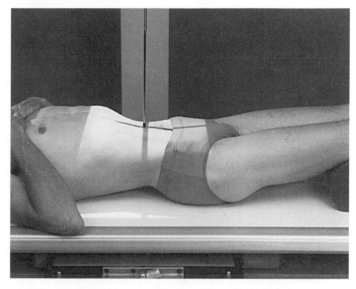

Figure 18-7 Supine urogram, AP projection.

23. True or False. The AP projection may be obtained with the patient either supine or upright.

24. True or False. Preliminary (scout) radiographs are most often obtained with the patient supine.

25. True or False. Postinjection radiographs are most often obtained with the patient upright.

26. What is the most likely purpose for obtaining an AP projection radiograph with the patient standing?

    a. To elongate the ureters
    b. To demonstrate ureteral reflux
    c. To demonstrate air–fluid levels
    d. To demonstrate the mobility of the kidneys

27. What adjustment in the supine patient's position can be made to help demonstrate the distal ends of the ureters?

    a. Place supports under the patient's knees.
    b. Place a support under the patient's lumbar region.
    c. Tilt the table and patient 15 to 20 degrees Trendelenburg.
    d. Position a compression band around the patient's abdomen.

28. What should be done to reduce the lordotic curvature when performing the AP projection with the patient recumbent?

    a. Place supports under the patient's knees.
    b. Tilt the table and patient 10 to 15 degrees Trendelenburg.
    c. Position a compression band around the patient's abdomen.

29. Which procedure should be performed if the bladder is not seen in the AP projection to demonstrate the entire urinary system?

    a. Center the IR to the level of L3.
    b. Direct the central ray 10 to 15 degrees cephalically.
    c. Make a separate AP projection radiograph of the bladder.
    d. Tilt the table and patient 10 to 15 degrees Trendelenburg.

30. Why is it desirable to include the area below the pubic symphysis for older male patients?

    a. To demonstrate distal ureters
    b. To demonstrate ureteral reflux
    c. To demonstrate the prostate region
    d. To demonstrate urinary bladder calculi

31. If a device is used for ureteral compression, to which level of the patient should it be centered?

    a. L1 to L3
    b. At the level of the ASIS
    c. 2 inches (5 cm) above the iliac crests
    d. 1 inch (2.5 cm) above the superior border of the pubic symphysis

32. Identify each lettered structure shown in Fig. 18-8.

    A. _____

    B. _____

    C. _____

    D. _____

    E. _____

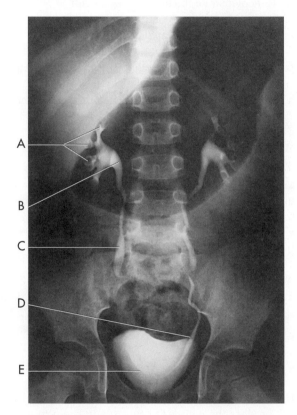

Figure 18-8 AP projection of the urinary system.

Questions 33 through 38 pertain to *AP oblique projections.* Examine Fig. 18-9 as you answer the following questions.

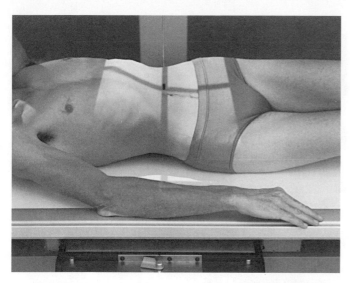

Figure 18-9 Urogram, AP oblique projection (RPO position).

33. Into which position should the patient be placed when beginning to position for either type of AP oblique projection?

    a. Prone
    b. Supine
    c. Lateral recumbent

34. When performing the AP oblique projection (right posterior oblique [RPO] position), which kidney will be parallel with the plane of the image receptor?

    a. Left
    b. Right

35. Approximately how many degrees should the patient be rotated from the supine position to an oblique position to demonstrate renal and urinary structures?

    a. 10 degrees
    b. 20 degrees
    c. 30 degrees
    d. 40 degrees

36. Which structure should be centered to the grid for the AP oblique projection (left posterior oblique [LPO] position)?

    a. Left kidney
    b. Right kidney
    c. Vertebral column

37. To which level of the patient should the image receptor (IR) be centered?

    a. L3
    b. Iliac crests
    c. Anterior superior iliac crests
    d. Pubic symphysis

38. Where should the central ray enter the patient?

    a. 2 inches lateral to the midline on the elevated side
    b. 2 inches lateral to the midline on the dependent side
    c. Centered to the midline 2 inches below the iliac crests

Items 39 through 43 pertain to the *lateral projection (lateral recumbent position)*. Examine Fig. 18-10 as you answer the following items.

Items 44 through 50 pertain to the *lateral projection (dorsal decubitus position)*. Examine Fig. 18-11 as you answer the following items.

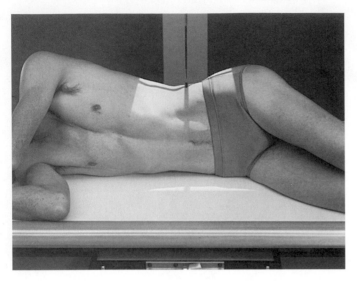

Figure 18-10 Urogram, lateral projection.

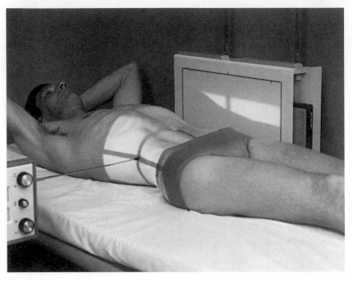

Figure 18-11 Urogram, lateral projection (dorsal decubitus position).

39. Which plane of the body should be centered to the grid?

_____

40. Describe how the patient's arms and hands should be placed.

41. Which areas of the patient should be examined to ensure that the patient is not rotated?

42. The exposure should be made at the end of

_____ (inspiration or expiration).

43. Exposure factors should produce a _____ (long or short) scale of contrast.

44. The dorsal decubitus position requires that the patient be

_____ (prone or supine).

45. The long axis of the IR should be centered to the

_____ plane.

46. Which area of the patient should be closest to the grid?
    a. Side
    b. Anterior
    c. Posterior

47. To which level of the patient should the image receptor be centered?
    a. L3
    b. Iliac crests
    c. Anterior superior iliac spines
    d. Pubic symphysis

48. True or False. Only male patients should have gonadal shielding for this type of projection.

49. True or False. The exposure should be made at the end of inspiration.

50. True or False. The central ray should be directed horizontal and perpendicular to the center of the image receptor.

Exercise 2: Retrograde Urography

Instructions: Retrograde urography is a radiographic procedure that demonstrates certain urinary structures. This exercise pertains to retrograde urography. Provide a short answer, select from a list, or choose true or false (explaining any statement you believe to be false) for each item.

Examine Fig. 18-12 as you answer the following items about retrograde urography.

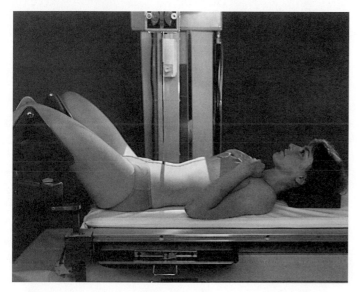

Figure 18-12 Patient positioned on the table for retrograde urography.

1. True or False. Retrograde urography differs from excretory urography in that the contrast medium is injected directly into the kidney by means of a percutaneous injection through the skin.

2. True or False. Retrograde urography is performed on a regular x-ray table.

3. At the beginning of the retrograde urographic examination, the patient should be placed in the modified _____ position.
   a. prone
   b. upright
   c. lithotomy
   d. lateral recumbent

4. Which IR size should be used for urograms of the typical adult?
   a. 18 × 24 cm
   b. 24 × 30 cm
   c. 35 × 43 cm

5. Who should inject the contrast medium?
   a. Urologist
   b. Radiologist
   c. Radiographer

6. Describe how a kidney function test can be performed during retrograde urography.

7. List the three AP projection radiographs that usually comprise a retrograde urographic examination.

8. Why might the head of the x-ray table be lowered 10 to 15 degrees during the retrograde pyelography procedure?

9. Which retrograde urographic radiograph sometimes requires that the head of the table be elevated 35 to 40 degrees?
   a. Pyelogram
   b. Ureterogram
   c. Preliminary radiograph showing catheter insertion

10. After necessary AP projections are made, which oblique positions are often used for oblique projections?
    a. RPO and LPO
    b. RPO and LAO
    c. RAO and LPO
    d. RAO and LAO

Exercise 3: Retrograde Cystography

Instructions: Projections obtained during retrograde cystography often include an AP projection, both AP oblique projections (RPO and LPO positions), and a lateral projection. This exercise pertains to those projections. Fill in missing words or provide a short answer for each item.

1. Describe how the contrast medium is introduced into the patient for retrograde cystography.

Questions 2 through 11 pertain to *AP axial* or *posteroanterior (PA) axial projections.* Examine Fig. 18-13 as you answer the following questions.

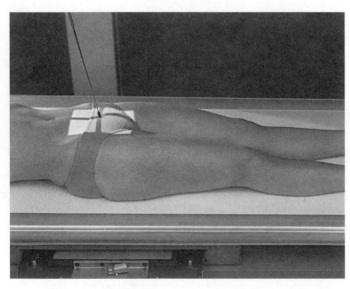

Figure 18-13 AP axial bladder.

2. For the typical adult, which size IR should be used to demonstrate the bladder, and how should it be placed in the IR holder?

   a. 18 × 24 cm; crosswise
   b. 18 × 24 cm; lengthwise
   c. 24 × 30 cm; crosswise
   d. 24 × 30 cm; lengthwise

3. Which structures are sometimes better demonstrated with the head of the table lowered 15 to 20 degrees?

   a. Prostate gland and urethra
   b. Lower (distal) ends of the ureters
   c. Upper (proximal) ends of the ureters

4. Why should patients in the supine position extend the lower limbs?

   a. To demonstrate ureteral reflux
   b. To retard the excretion of opacified urine from the bladder
   c. To enable the lumbar lordotic curve to arch the pelvis enough to tilt the pubic bones inferiorly

5. Which breathing instructions should be given to the patient?

   a. Slow breathing
   b. Suspend breathing after expiration
   c. Suspend breathing after inspiration

6. To demonstrate the bladder during cystography, how many degrees and in which direction should the central ray be directed for the AP axial projection?

   a. 5 degrees caudal
   b. 5 degrees cephalic
   c. 10 to 15 degrees caudal
   d. 10 to 15 degrees cephalic

7. To which level of the patient should the central ray enter for the AP axial projection?

   a. The iliac crests
   b. 2 inches (5 cm) above the upper border of the pubic symphysis
   c. 2 inches (5 cm) below the upper border of the pubic symphysis

8. How should the patient be positioned to best demonstrate the prostate?

   a. Prone
   b. Supine
   c. Upright
   d. Lateral recumbent

9. How should the central ray be directed to best demonstrate the prostate?

   a. Caudally
   b. Cephalically
   c. Perpendicularly

10. If minor reflux is present at the bladder, what other structures most likely will be demonstrated?

    a. Both kidneys
    b. Distal ureters
    c. Prostate gland

11. How should the pubic bones be demonstrated in the image of the AP axial projection?

    a. They should superimpose both the bladder neck and the proximal urethra.
    b. They should be projected above both the bladder neck and the proximal urethra.
    c. They should be projected below both the bladder neck and the proximal urethra.

Items 12 through 16 pertain to *AP oblique projections.* Examine Fig. 18-14 as you answer the following items.

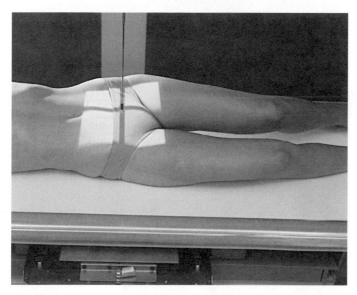

Figure 18-14 Retrograde cystogram, AP oblique projection (RPO position).

12. In which position should the patient be placed?

    a. Semiprone
    b. Semisupine
    c. Lateral recumbent

13. How should the patient's uppermost thigh be positioned to prevent it from superimposing the bladder in AP oblique projections?

    a. Crossed over the other thigh
    b. Flexed and placed at right angles to the abdomen
    c. Extended and abducted enough to prevent its superimposition on the bladder area

14. How many degrees should the patient be rotated for AP oblique projections?

    a. 10 to 15
    b. 20 to 30
    c. 40 to 60

15. From the following list, circle the two ways that the central ray can be directed for AP oblique projections.

    a. Perpendicularly
    b. 10 degrees caudally
    c. 10 degrees cephalically
    d. 20 degrees caudally
    e. 20 degrees cephalically

16. With reference to the pubic bones, where should the bladder neck be seen in the AP oblique projection radiograph, RPO position?

    a. Above
    b. Below
    c. To the left side
    d. To the right side

Questions 17 through 20 pertain to the *lateral projection.* Examine Fig. 18-15 as you answer the following questions.

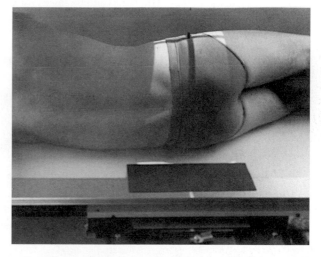

Figure 18-15 Cystogram, lateral projection.

17. Which body position should be used for the lateral projection for cystography?

    a. Upright lateral
    b. Lateral recumbent
    c. Ventral decubitus (prone)
    d. Dorsal decubitus (supine)

18. Where should the image receptor be centered for the lateral projection?

    a. At the level of the iliac crests
    b. At the level of the pubic symphysis
    c. 2 inches (5 cm) above the iliac crests
    d. 2 inches (5 cm) above the pubic symphysis

19. How should the central ray be directed?

    a. Horizontally
    b. Perpendicularly
    c. Angled caudally
    d. Angled cephalically

20. Which imaged structures can determine whether the patient was rotated from the lateral position?

    a. Lumbar vertebrae
    b. Crests of the ilia
    c. Hips and femora

Exercise 4: Male Cystourethrography

Instructions: This exercise pertains to male cystourethrography. Provide a short answer, select from a list, or choose true or false (explaining any statement you believe to be false) for each item. Examine Fig. 18-16 as you answer the following items.

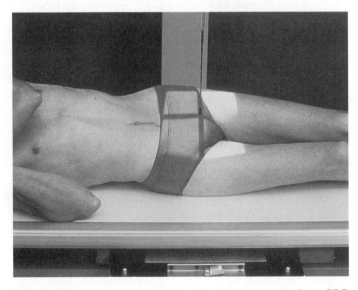

Figure 18-16 Cystourethrogram, AP oblique projection RPO position).

1. Define cystourethrography.

2. Describe how the contrast medium is introduced into the urinary structures of interest.

3. After the contrast medium is introduced into the patient, in which two positions can the patient be placed to demonstrate urinary structures?

    a. RAO and LAO
    b. RAO and LPO
    c. RPO and LAO
    d. RPO and LPO

4. How many degrees should the patient be rotated for the desired oblique projection?

    a. 15 to 20 degrees
    b. 25 to 30 degrees
    c. 35 to 40 degrees

5. To which level of the patient should the IR be centered?

    a. Crests of the ilia
    b. Anterior superior iliac spines
    c. 2 inches (5 cm) above the superior border of the pubic symphysis
    d. Superior border of the pubic symphysis

6. True or False. To ensure adequate coverage, the IR should be placed lengthwise.

7. True or False. To ensure that the entire urethra is filled, the exposure should be made while the physician is injecting the contrast medium.

8. True or False. After the bladder is filled with contrast medium, the voiding film can be exposed with the patient in either a posterior oblique or an upright position.

9. True or False. The radiation field should be large enough to include the entire urinary system on all radiographs.

10. Identify each lettered structure shown in Fig. 18-17.

A. _____

B. _____

C. _____

D. _____

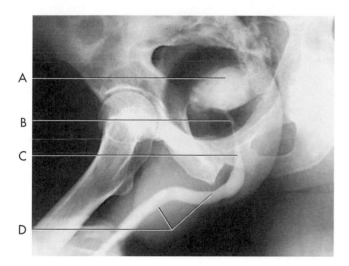

Figure 18-17 Cystourethrogram, AP oblique projection (RPO position).

Exercise 5: Identifying Urinary System Radiographs

Instructions: Identify each of the following radiographs by selecting the best choice from the list provided for each image.

1. Fig. 18-18:
   a. Excretory urogram, AP projection
   b. Retrograde urogram, AP projection
   c. Excretory cystogram, AP projection
   d. Preliminary (scout) radiograph, AP projection

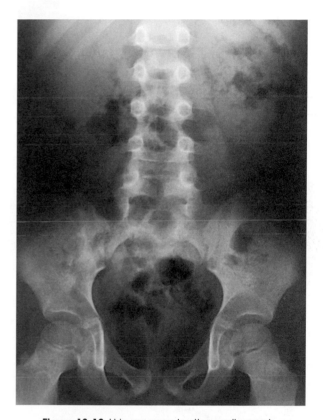

Figure 18-18 Urinary examination radiograph.

2. Fig. 18-19:

   a. Excretory urogram, AP projection
   b. Retrograde urogram, AP projection
   c. Excretory cystogram, AP projection
   d. Preliminary (scout) radiograph, AP projection

3. Fig. 18-20:

   a. Excretory urogram, AP projection
   b. Retrograde urogram, AP projection
   c. Excretory cystogram, AP projection
   d. Preliminary (scout) radiograph, AP projection

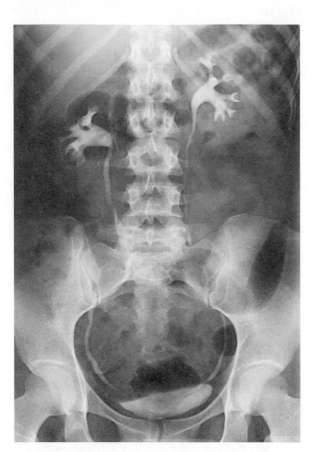

Figure 18-19 Urinary examination radiograph.

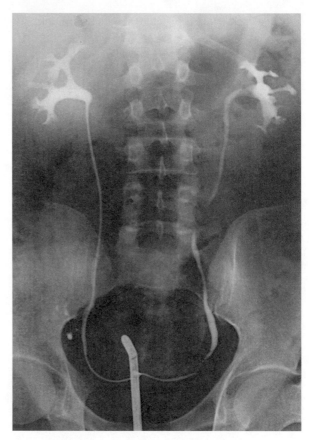

Figure 18-20 Urinary examination radiograph.

4. Fig. 18-21:

   a. Excretory urogram, AP oblique projection (LPO position)
   b. Excretory urogram, AP oblique projection (RPO position)
   c. Retrograde cystogram, AP oblique projection (LPO position)
   d. Retrograde cystogram, AP oblique projection (RPO position)

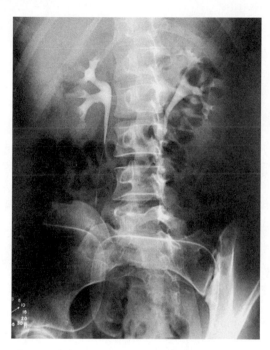

Figure 18-21 Urinary examination radiograph.

5. Fig. 18-22:

   a. Urogram, lateral projection
   b. Urogram, left lateral decubitus
   c. Excretory urogram, AP oblique projection (RPO position)
   d. Excretory urogram, AP oblique projection (LPO position)

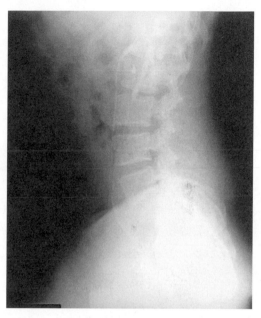

Figure 18-22 Urinary examination radiograph.

6. Fig. 18-23:

   a. Prevoiding filled bladder, AP projection
   b. Postvoiding emptied bladder, AP projection
   c. Retrograde cystogram, AP oblique projection (RPO position)
   d. Injection cystourethrogram, AP oblique projection (RPO position)

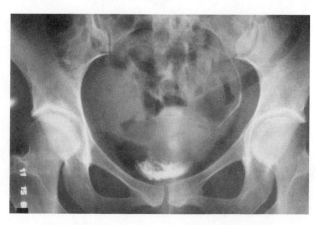

Figure 18-23 Urinary examination radiograph.

7. Fig. 18-24:

   a. Prevoiding filled bladder, AP projection

   b. Postvoiding emptied bladder, AP projection

   c. Retrograde cystogram, AP oblique projection (RPO position)

   d. Injection cystourethrogram, AP oblique projection (RPO position)

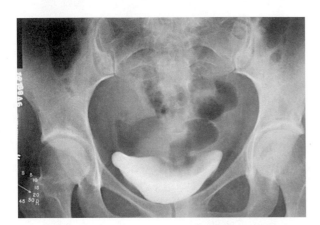

Figure 18-24 Urinary examination radiograph.

8. Fig. 18-25:

   a. Excretory cystogram, AP projection

   b. Retrograde cystogram, AP projection

   c. Postvoiding emptied bladder, AP projection

   d. Retrograde cystogram, AP oblique projection (RPO position)

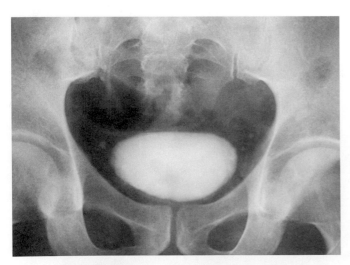

Figure 18-25 Urinary examination radiograph.

9. Fig. 18-26:

   a. Excretory cystogram, AP projection

   b. Retrograde cystogram, AP projection

   c. Postvoiding emptied bladder, AP projection

   d. Retrograde cystogram, AP oblique projection (RPO position)

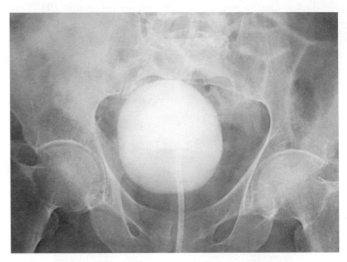

Figure 18-26 Urinary examination radiograph.

10. Fig. 18-27

   a. Excretory cystogram, AP projection

   b. Retrograde cystogram, AP projection

   c. Postvoiding emptied bladder, AP projection

   d. Retrograde cystogram, AP oblique projection (RPO position)

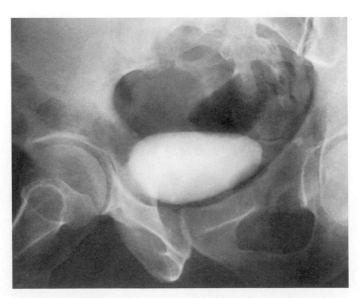

Figure 18-27 Urinary examination radiograph.

Self-Test: Anatomy and Positioning of the Urinary System

Instructions: Answer the following questions by selecting the best choice.

1. Which renal structure filters the blood?

   a. Glomerulus
   b. Major calyx
   c. Efferent arteriole
   d. Afferent arteriole

2. Which urinary excretory duct conveys urine from the bladder to outside the body?

   a. Ureter
   b. Urethra
   c. Efferent arteriole
   d. Afferent arteriole

3. Which body organ filters blood and produces urine as a by-product of waste material?

   a. Liver
   b. Spleen
   c. Kidney
   d. Pancreas

4. At which vertebral level is the superior border of the kidneys usually found?

   a. T10
   b. T12
   c. L2
   d. L4

5. What is the name of the opening on the medial border of a kidney?

   a. Pole
   b. Base
   c. Apex
   d. Hilum

6. Which of the following is an excretory examination used to demonstrate the upper urinary tract?

   a. Cystourethrography
   b. Retrograde urography
   c. Intravenous urography
   d. Retrograde cystography

7. Which examination has the ability to produce a radiographic image demonstrating renal cortical tissue well saturated with contrast medium?

   a. Cystourethrography
   b. Retrograde urography
   c. Intravenous urography
   d. Retrograde cystography

8. Which projection best demonstrates the mobility of the kidneys?

   a. AP projection with the patient supine
   b. AP projection with the patient upright
   c. Lateral projection with the patient lateral recumbent
   d. Lateral projection with the patient supine (dorsal decubitus position)

9. In intravenous urography, what is the purpose of applying compression pads over the distal ends of both ureters?

   a. To demonstrate ureteral reflux
   b. To demonstrate the mobility of the kidneys
   c. To retard the flow of opacified urine into the bladder
   d. To retard the flow of opacified urine from the bladder

10. Which of the following is *not* a reason for obtaining a scout radiograph with the patient recumbent for excretory urography?

    a. To evaluate exposure factors
    b. To demonstrate urinary calculi
    c. To determine the location of the kidneys
    d. To demonstrate the mobility of the kidneys

11. For excretory urography, what should an adult patient do just before getting on the examination table?

    a. Empty the bladder.
    b. Remove all jewelry.
    c. Drink 12 ounces of cold water.
    d. Drink 12 ounces of carbonated beverage.

12. What is the purpose of obtaining an AP projection radiograph of the kidneys 30 seconds after the bolus injection of a contrast medium in excretory urography?

    a. To demonstrate ureteral reflux
    b. To demonstrate opacified renal cortex
    c. To demonstrate opacified renal arteries
    d. To demonstrate the mobility of the kidneys

13. What is the purpose of tilting the patient and table 15 to 20 degrees Trendelenburg for the AP projection during excretory urography?

    a. To demonstrate distal ureters
    b. To demonstrate opacified renal cortex
    c. To demonstrate the base of the bladder
    d. To demonstrate the mobility of the kidneys

14. How many degrees should the patient be rotated for posterior (AP) oblique projections during excretory urography?

    a. 15
    b. 30
    c. 45
    d. 60

15. For intravenous urography of a child, what should the patient be given when the scout radiograph shows an excessive amount of intestinal gas overlying the kidneys?

    a. A laxative
    b. A cleansing enema
    c. 12 ounces of iced water
    d. 12 ounces of carbonated beverage

16. Which examination requires that the patient be placed on a special urographic–radiographic examination table?

    a. Cystourethrography
    b. Retrograde urography
    c. Intravenous urography
    d. Retrograde cystography

17. Which renal structures are not demonstrated during retrograde urographic examinations?

    a. Ureters
    b. Nephrons
    c. Minor calyces
    d. Major calyces

18. In addition to the AP projection, which projection would most likely be included in the radiographs for retrograde urography?

    a. PA projection
    b. PA oblique projection
    c. AP oblique projection
    d. AP projection, lateral decubitus position

19. What is the purpose of tilting the table 10 to 15 degrees Trendelenburg for retrograde urography?

    a. To demonstrate the ureters
    b. To demonstrate the mobility of the kidneys
    c. To produce a nephrogram effect in the kidneys
    d. To prevent contrast medium from escaping the kidneys

20. What is the purpose of raising the head of the table 35 to 40 degrees for retrograde urography?

    a. To demonstrate the ureters
    b. To position the patient for catheterization
    c. To produce a nephrogram effect in the kidneys
    d. To prevent contrast medium from escaping the kidneys

21. Which condition would most likely be demonstrated during voiding cystography?

    a. Renal cyst
    b. Renal calculi
    c. Ureteral reflux
    d. Hydronephrosis

22. For the AP axial projection of the bladder, how many degrees and in which direction should the central ray be directed?

    a. 15 degrees caudal
    b. 15 degrees cephalic
    c. 25 degrees caudal
    d. 25 degrees cephalic

23. For retrograde cystography, which projection should be performed to demonstrate the anterior and posterior walls of the bladder?

    a. Upright AP projection
    b. Recumbent AP projection
    c. Direct lateral projection
    d. AP projection, lateral decubitus position

24. For cystourethrography with an adult male patient, to which level of the patient should the IR be centered?

    a. T12 vertebra
    b. L3 vertebra
    c. L5 vertebra
    d. Pubic symphysis

25. For cystourethrography with an adult male patient, which of the following should be used to obtain a radiograph while the patient is urinating?

    a. Recumbent PA projection
    b. Dorsal decubitus position
    c. Lateral decubitus position
    d. Recumbent AP oblique projection

CHAPTER 19

Reproductive System

SECTION 1

Anatomy of the Reproductive System

Exercise 1

Instructions: This exercise pertains to the anatomy of the female reproductive system. Identify structures, fill in missing words, provide a short answer, or match columns for each item.

1. Identify each lettered structure shown in Fig. 19-1.

A. _____

B. _____

C. _____

D. _____

E. _____

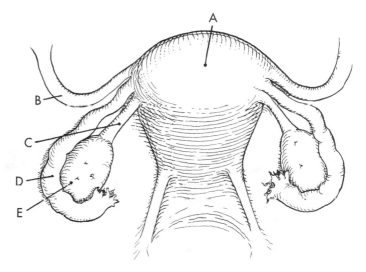

Figure 19-1 Superoposterior view of the uterus, ovaries, and uterine tubes.

2. Identify each lettered structure shown in Fig. 19-2.

A. _____   G. _____

B. _____   H. _____

C. _____   I. _____

D. _____   J. _____

E. _____   K. _____

F. _____   L. _____

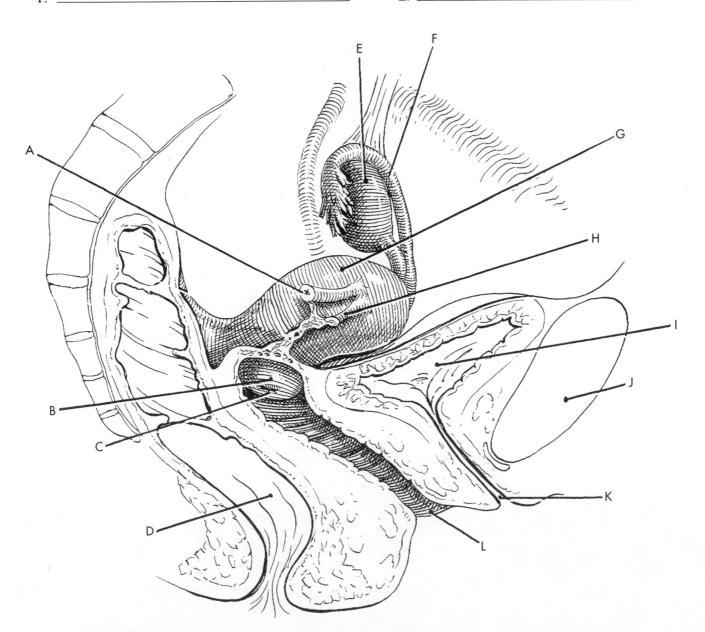

Figure 19-2 Sagittal section showing the relation of the internal genitalia to the surrounding structures.

3. The female gonads are called the _____.

4. Female reproductive cells are called _____.

5. The structure that conveys an ovum from a gonad to the uterus is the _____ tube.

6. The number of uterine tubes in the typical adult female is _____.

7. The pear-shaped muscular organ of the female reproductive system is the _____.

8. Name the four main parts of the uterus.

9. What part of the uterus is referred to as the neck?

10. Match the uterine structures in Column A with the definitions in Column B.

Column A	Column B
____ 1. Body	a. Superiormost portion
____ 2. Fundus	b. Cylindrical vaginal end
____ 3. Cervix	c. Mucosal lining of the uterine cavity
____ 4. Isthmus	d. Constricted area adjacent to the vaginal end
____ 5. Endometrium	e. Where ligaments attach the uterus within the pelvis

Exercise 2

Instructions: This exercise pertains to the anatomy of the male reproductive system. Identify structures or fill in missing words for each item.

1. Identify each lettered structure shown in Fig.19-3.

   A. _____

   B. _____

   C. _____

   D. _____

   E. _____

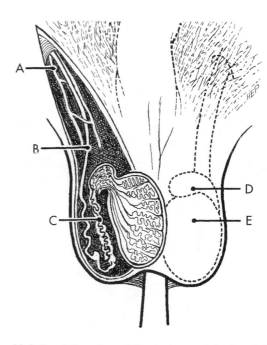

Figure 19-3 Frontal section of the testes and ductus deferens.

2. Identify each lettered structure in Fig. 19-4.

A. _____

B. _____

C. _____

D. _____

E. _____

F. _____

G. _____

3. Identify each lettered structure shown in Fig. 19-5.

A. _____

B. _____

C. _____

D. _____

E. _____

F. _____

G. _____

H. _____

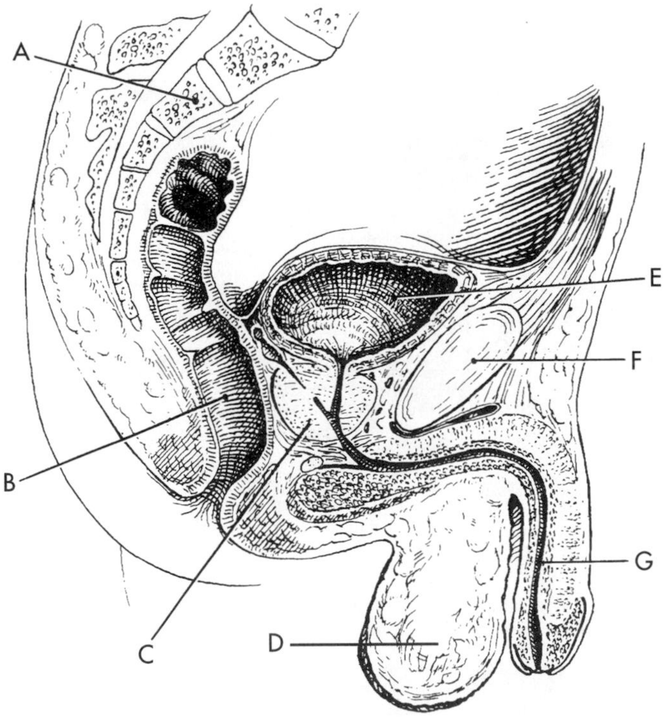

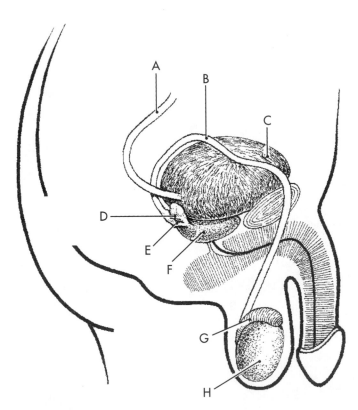

Figure 19-4 Sagittal section showing the male genital system.

Figure 19-5 Sagittal section through the male pelvis.

4. The male gonads are called the _____.

5. Male reproductive cells are called _____.

6. The oblong structure attached to each testicle is the

   _____.

7. The excretory channel that allows male germ cells to pass

   from a gonad to the urethra is the _____

   _____.

8. The union of the ductus deferens and the seminal vesicle

   duct forms the _____ duct.

9. The accessory genital organ that is composed of muscular

   and glandular tissues is the _____.

10. The ducts from the prostate open into the proximal portion

    of the _____.

SECTION 2

Radiography of the Reproductive System

Exercise 1: Radiography of the Female Reproductive System

Instructions: Although other imaging modalities have reduced the demand for radiographic examinations of the female reproductive system, some facilities still radiographically demonstrate female reproductive structures. This exercise pertains to radiographic visualization of the female reproductive system. Match columns of relevant information or select the correct answer from a list for each item.

1. Match each radiographic examination from Column A with the type of patient from Column B who is most likely to undergo that type of examination.

   Column A

   _____ 1. Fetography

   _____ 2. Pelvimetry

   _____ 3. Vaginography

   _____ 4. Placentography

   _____ 5. Pelvic pneumography

   _____ 6. Hysterosalpingography

   Column B

   a. Pregnant patient

   b. Nongravid patient

2. Match the descriptions in Column A with the corresponding type of examination in Column B. Some descriptions may have more than one examination associated with them. Examinations will be used more than once.

Column A

_____ 1. Determines pelvic diameters

_____ 2. Uses a Colcher-Sussman ruler

_____ 3. Helps determine placenta previa

_____ 4. Requires a gaseous contrast agent

_____ 5. Requires the use of a contrast agent

_____ 6. Requires a radiopaque contrast agent

_____ 7. Investigates the patency of uterine tubes

_____ 8. Largely replaced by diagnostic ultrasound

_____ 9. Performed to demonstrate a fetus in utero

_____ 10. Introduces a contrast agent into the vaginal canal

_____ 11. Introduces a contrast agent through a uterine cannula

_____ 12. Introduces a contrast agent directly into the peritoneal cavity

_____ 13. Should be performed about 10 days after the onset of menstruation

_____ 14. Performed to determine the of size, shape, and position the uterus and uterine tubes

_____ 15. Performed to demonstrate congenital abnormalities of the muscular structure that extends from the cervix to the external genitalia

Column B

a. Fetography

b. Pelvimetry

c. Vaginography

d. Placentography

e. Pelvic pneumography

f. Hysterosalpingography

3. Figs. 19-6 through 19-10 are representative examinations of the female reproductive system. Examine the images, then select the best answer from the list provided for each image.

i. Fig. 19-6:
   a. Pelvimetry
   b. Vaginography
   c. Pelvic pneumography
   d. Hysterosalpingography

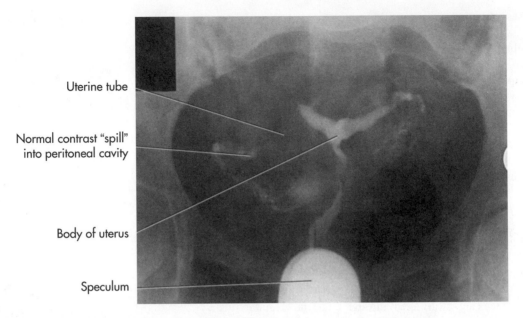

Uterine tube

Normal contrast "spill" into peritoneal cavity

Body of uterus

Speculum

Figure 19-6 Radiograph of the female reproductive system.

ii. Fig. 19-7:
   a. Fetography
   b. Vaginography
   c. Pelvic pneumography
   d. Hysterosalpingography

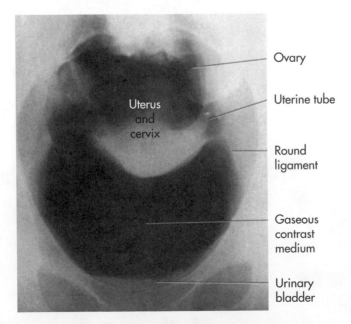

Uterus and cervix

Ovary

Uterine tube

Round ligament

Gaseous contrast medium

Urinary bladder

Figure 19-7 Radiograph of the female reproductive system.

iii. Fig. 19-8:
   a. Pelvimetry
   b. Vaginography
   c. Pelvic pneumography
   d. Hysterosalpingography

iv. Fig. 19-9:
   a. Pelvimetry
   b. Fetography
   c. Placentography
   d. Hysterosalpingography

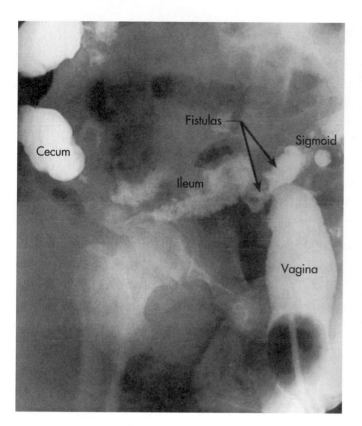

Figure 19-8 Radiograph of the female reproductive system.

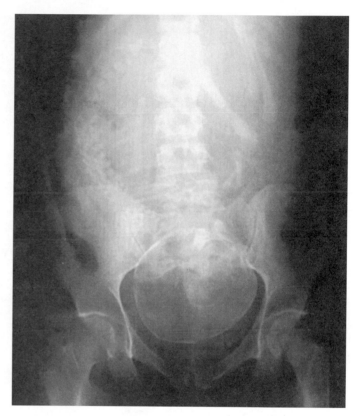

Figure 19-9 Radiograph of the female reproductive system.

v. Fig. 19-10:
   a. Pelvimetry
   b. Fetography
   c. Placentography
   d. Pelvic pneumography

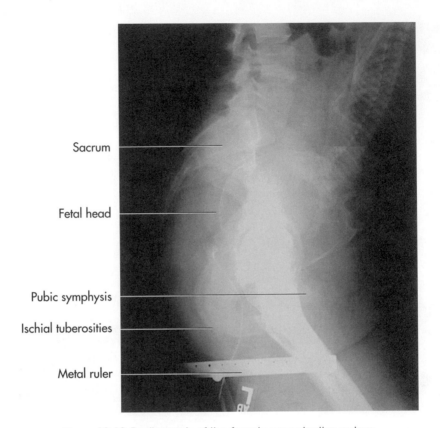

Sacrum

Fetal head

Pubic symphysis

Ischial tuberosities

Metal ruler

Figure 19-10 Radiograph of the female reproductive system.

Exercise 2: Radiography of the Male Reproductive System

Instructions: Although the demand for radiographic visualization of the male reproductive system has greatly decreased in recent years because of advances with diagnostic ultrasound, some facilities still radiographically demonstrate male reproductive structures. This exercise pertains to radiographic visualization of the male reproductive system. Provide a short answer for each question.

1. What type of contrast medium is used for radiographic examination of the seminal ducts?

2. Why might a radiolucent contrast medium be injected into the scrotum for epididymography?

3. What accessory organ of the male reproductive system can be radiographically examined?

4. What body position is preferred for radiography of the prostate? Explain why.

5. For posteroanterior (PA) projections of the prostate, how many degrees and in which direction should the central ray be directed?

Self-Test: Reproductive System

Instructions: Answer the following questions by selecting the best choice.

1. Which structures are part of the female reproductive system?
   a. Ovaries, uterus, and fallopian tubes
   b. Ovaries, testes, and ductus deferens
   c. Epididymis, uterus, and fallopian tubes
   d. Epididymis, testes, and ductus deferens

2. Which part of the uterus is most superior?
   a. Body
   b. Cervix
   c. Fundus
   d. Isthmus

3. Which structure conveys female reproductive cells from a gonad to the uterus?
   a. Urethra
   b. Uterine tube
   c. Ductus deferens
   d. Ejaculatory duct

4. Which structure produces female reproductive cells?
   a. Ovary
   b. Uterus
   c. Testicle
   d. Epididymis

5. Which structure produces spermatozoa?
   a. Ovary
   b. Testicle
   c. Prostate
   d. Epididymis

6. Which structure conveys male reproductive cells from a gonad to the urethra?
   a. Uterine tube
   b. Fallopian tube
   c. Ductus deferens
   d. Ejaculatory duct

7. Which structure is attached to each male gonad?
   a. Urethra
   b. Prostate
   c. Epididymis
   d. Ejaculatory duct

8. Which examination can be performed on a pregnant patient?
   a. Fetography
   b. Prostatography
   c. Pelvic pneumography
   d. Hysterosalpingography

9. Which examination can be performed on a nongravid patient?
   a. Fetography
   b. Pelvimetry
   c. Placentography
   d. Hysterosalpingography

10. Which examination introduces contrast medium through a uterine cannula?
    a. Fetography
    b. Pelvimetry
    c. Vaginography
    d. Hysterosalpingography

11. Which examination is performed to verify the patency of uterine tubes?
    a. Fetography
    b. Pelvimetry
    c. Placentography
    d. Hysterosalpingography

12. Which examination determines pelvic diameters?
    a. Fetography
    b. Pelvimetry
    c. Placentography
    d. Hysterosalpingography

13. Which type of contrast medium is preferred for hysterosalpingography?
    a. Oily viscous
    b. Water-soluble
    c. Barium sulfate

14. When should a hysterosalpingographic examination be performed?
    a. After the first trimester
    b. During the first trimester
    c. 10 days after the onset of menstruation
    d. 10 days before the onset of menstruation

15. Which projection is preferred for prostatography?
    a. AP axial
    b. PA axial
    c. Lateral
    d. AP oblique (right posterior oblique [RPO] position)

CHAPTER 20

Skull

SECTION 1

Osteology of the Skull

Exercise 1

Instructions: This exercise pertains to the osteology of the skull. Identify structures for each illustration.

1. Identify each lettered structure shown in Fig. 20-1.

A. _____

B. _____

C. _____

D. _____

E. _____

F. _____

G. _____

H. _____

I. _____

J. _____

K. _____

L. _____

M. _____

N. _____

O. _____

P. _____

Q. _____

R. _____

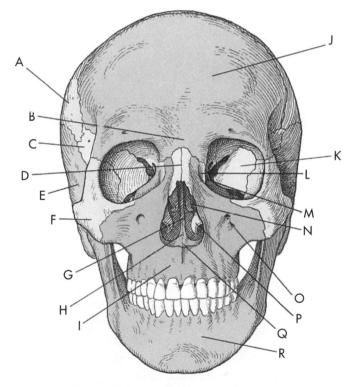

Figure 20-1 Anterior aspect of the skull.

2. Identify each lettered structure shown in Fig. 20-2.

A. _____

B. _____

C. _____

D. _____

E. _____

F. _____

G. _____

H. _____

I. _____

J. _____

K. _____

L. _____

M. _____ (fontanel)

N. _____ (suture)

O. _____

P. _____ (suture)

Q. _____ (fontanel)

R. _____ (suture)

S. _____

T. _____

U. _____

V. _____

W. _____

X. _____

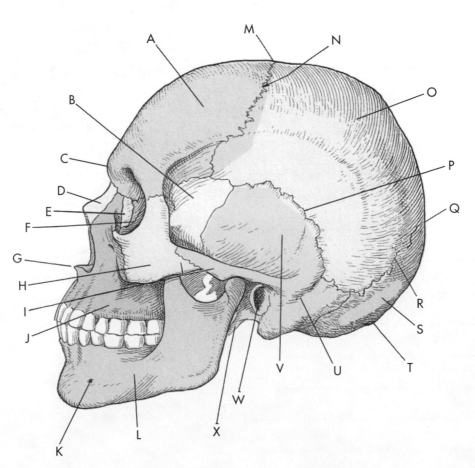

Figure 20-2 Lateral aspect of the skull.

3. Identify each lettered structure shown in Fig. 20-3.

A. _____   L. _____

B. _____   M. _____

C. _____   N. _____

D. _____   O. _____

E. _____   P. _____

F. _____   Q. _____

G. _____   R. _____

H. _____   S. _____

I. _____   T. _____

J. _____   U. _____

K. _____   V. _____

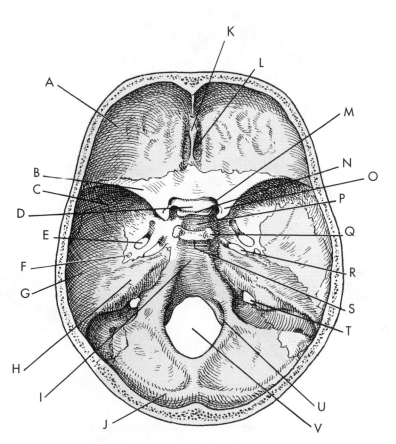

Figure 20-3 Superior aspect of the cranial base.

4. Identify each lettered structure shown in Fig. 20-4.

A. _____

B. _____

C. _____

D. _____

E. _____

F. _____

G. _____

H. _____

I. _____

J. _____

K. _____

L. _____

M. _____

N. _____

O. _____

P. _____

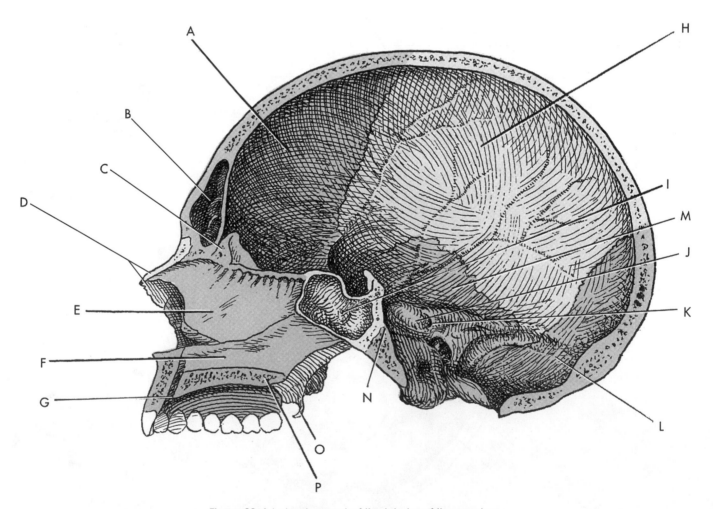

Figure 20-4 Lateral aspect of the interior of the cranium.

5. Identify each lettered structure shown in Fig. 20-5.

A. _____

B. _____

C. _____

D. _____

E. _____

F. _____

G. _____

6. Identify each lettered structure shown in Fig. 20-6.

A. _____

B. _____

C. _____

D. _____

E. _____

F. _____

G. _____

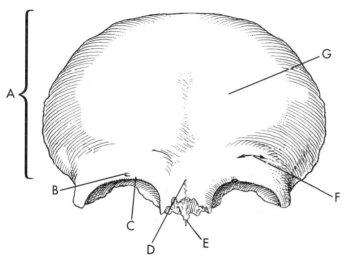

Figure 20-5 Anterior aspect of the frontal bone.

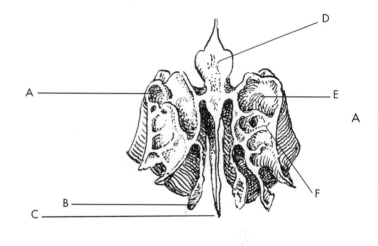

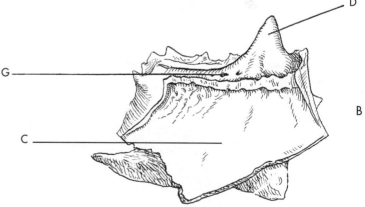

Figure 20-6 Two illustrations of the ethmoid bone: **A,** The anterior aspect. **B,** The lateral aspect with the labyrinth removed.

7. Identify the four angles and the four articulating borders of the left parietal bone shown in Fig. 20-7.

A. Articulates with the _____ bone

B. _____ angle

C. Articulates with the _____ bone

D. _____ angle

E. _____ angle

F. Articulates with the _____ bone

G. _____ angle

H. Articulates with the _____ bone

8. Identify each lettered structure shown in Fig. 20-8.

A. _____

B. _____

C. _____

D. _____

E. _____

F. _____

G. _____

H. _____

I. _____

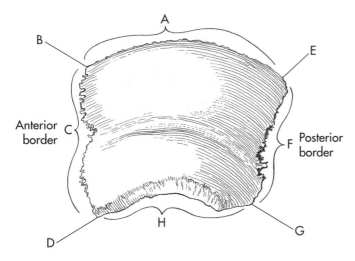

Figure 20-7 External surface of the left parietal bone.

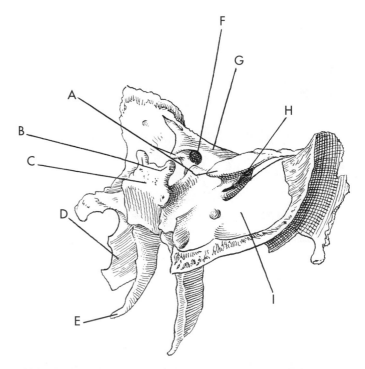

Figure 20-8 Oblique view of the upper and lateroposterior aspects of the sphenoid bone.

9. Identify each lettered structure shown in Fig. 20-9.

A. _____

B. _____

C. _____

D. _____

E. _____

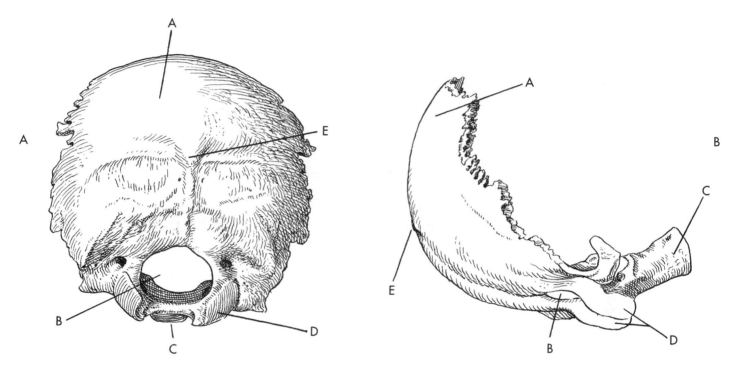

Figure 20-9 Two illustrations of the occipital bone: **A,** The external surface. **B,** The lateroinferior surface.

10. Identify each lettered structure shown in Fig. 20-10.

A. _____   F. _____

B. _____   G. _____

C. _____   H. _____

D. _____   I. _____

E. _____

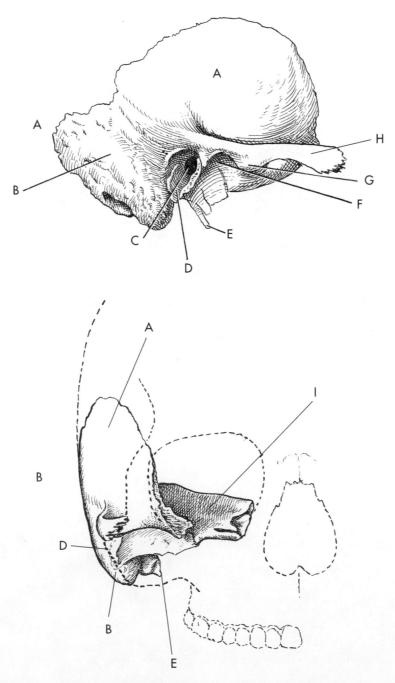

Figure 20-10 Two illustrations of the temporal bone: **A,** The lateral aspect. **B,** The anterior aspect in relation to the surrounding structures.

11. Identify each lettered structure shown in Fig. 20-11.

A. _____

B. _____

C. _____

D. _____

E. _____

F. _____

G. _____

H. _____

I. _____

J. _____

K. _____

L. _____

M. _____

N. _____

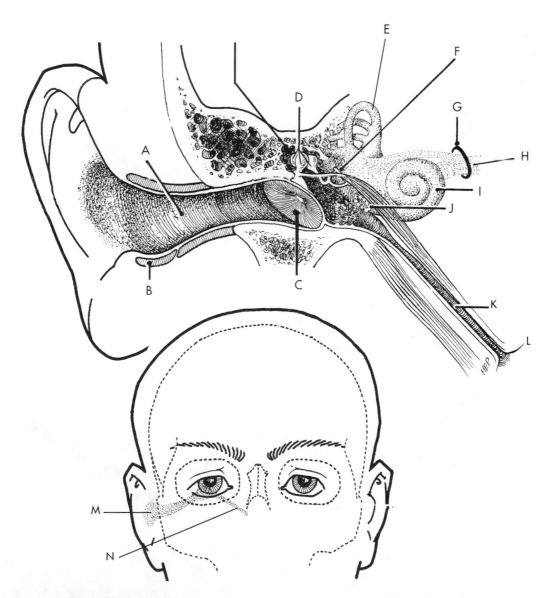

Figure 20-11 Frontal section through the right ear showing the internal structures.

12. Identify each lettered structure shown in Fig. 20-12.

A. _____

B. _____

C. _____

D. _____

E. _____

F. _____

G. _____

H. _____

I. _____

J. _____

K. _____

13. Identify each lettered structure shown in Fig. 20-13.

A. _____

B. _____

C. _____

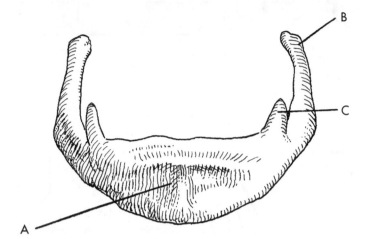

Figure 20-13 Anterior aspect of the hyoid.

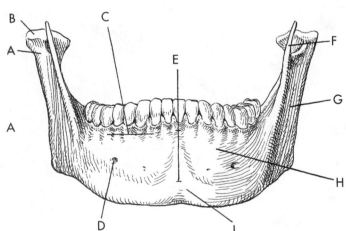

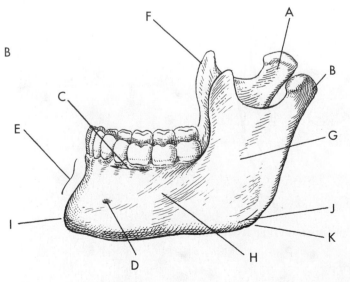

Figure 20-12 Two illustrations of the mandible: **A,** The anterior aspect. **B,** The lateral aspect.

Exercise 2

Instructions: Use the following clues to complete the crossword puzzle. All answers refer to the skull.

ACROSS

1. Perpendicular _____
4. Midpoint of the frontonasal suture
5. This bone has wings
7. Vertical part of the frontal bone
8. _____ galli
9. Number of cranial bones
12. Densest part of the cranial floor
13. Articulates frontal bone with parietals
16. Fibrous cranial joint
19. Anterior fontanel
20. Posterior fontanel
21. Forms top of the cranium
22. Posterior part of the skull
23. Eyebrow arches

DOWN

1. Inferior sphenoidal process
2. Sphenoidal endocrine
3. _____ turcica
5. Lateral suture
6. Long and narrow skull
10. Average skull
11. Smooth frontal elevation
14. Posterior to the nasal bones
15. Ear bone
17. Where occipital bone joins parietals
18. Forehead bone
19. Anteroinferior occipital part

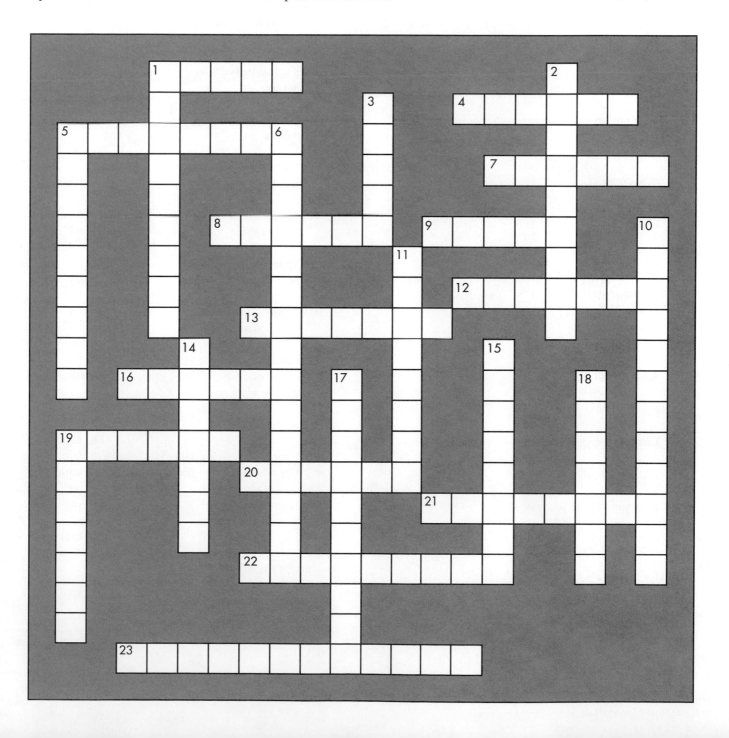

Exercise 3

Instructions: Match the structures (Column A) with the cranial bones on which they are found (Column B).

Column A   Column B

____ 1. Nasion   a. Frontal

____ 2. Glabella   b. Ethmoid

____ 3. Four angles   c. Parietal

____ 4. Lesser wing   d. Sphenoid

____ 5. Greater wing   e. Temporal

____ 6. Two condyles   f. Occipital

____ 7. Crista galli

____ 8. Sella turcica

____ 9. Foramen magnum

____ 10. Cribriform plate

____ 11. Mastoid process

____ 12. Basilar portion

____ 13. Petrous portion

____ 14. Pterygoid hamulus

____ 15. Zygomatic process

____ 16. Supraorbital margin

____ 17. Perpendicular plate

____ 18. Lateral pterygoid process

____ 19. Anterior clinoid processes

____ 20. Posterior clinoid processes

Exercise 4

Instructions: Match the statements (Column A) with the facial bone terms to which they refer (Column B). Only one selection from Column B applies to each statement in Column A. Not all terms from Column B should be used.

Column A   Column B

____ 1. Cheekbone   a. Head

____ 2. Largest facial bone   b. Body

____ 3. Number of facial bones   c. Nasal

____ 4. Forms bridge of the   d. Hyoid
        nose
                                  e. Ramus
____ 5. Vertical mandibular
        portion   f. Vomer

____ 6. Found in the roof of the g. Gonion
        mouth
                                  h. Twelve
____ 7. Midpoint of the anterior
        nasal spine   i. Fourteen

____ 8. Articulating process of   j. Lacrimal
        the mandible
                                  k. Alveolar
____ 9. Spongy processes that
        hold the teeth   l. Condyle

____ 10. Anterior part of the   m. Zygoma
         mandibular ramus
                                  n. Palatine
____ 11. Landmark at the angle
         of the mandible   o. Maxillae

____ 12. Found in the medial   p. Coronoid
         walls of the orbits
                                  q. Mandible
____ 13. Forms the inferior por-
         tion of the nasal septum r. Acanthion

____ 14. Horseshoe-shaped   s. Inferior conchae
         mandibular portion
                                  t. Mental
____ 15. Thin, scroll-like bones   protuberance
         that extend horizontally
         inside nasal cavity

Exercise 5

Instructions: Match the pathology terms in Column A with the appropriate definition in Column B. Not all choices from Column B should be selected.

Column A

_____ 1. Sinusitis

_____ 2. Mastoiditis

_____ 3. TMJ syndrome

_____ 4. Basal fracture

_____ 5. Linear fracture

_____ 6. Tripod fracture

_____ 7. LeFort fracture

_____ 8. Blowout fracture

_____ 9. Depressed fracture

_____ 10. Contre-coup fracture

_____ 11. Osteoma

_____ 12. Metastases

_____ 13. Acoustic neuroma

_____ 14. Pituitary adenoma

_____ 15. Multiple myeloma

Column B

a. Tumor composed of bony tissue

b. Fracture of the floor of the orbit

c. Irregular or jagged fracture of the skull

d. Fracture located at the base of the skull

e. Dysfunction of the temporomandibular joint

f. Bilateral horizontal fractures of the maxillae

g. Inflammation of the mastoid antrum and air cells

h. Inflammation of the bone due to a pyogenic infection

i. Inflammation of one or more of the paranasal sinuses

j. Transfer of a cancerous lesion from one area to another

k. Tumor arising from the pituitary gland, usually in the anterior lobe

l. Benign tumor arising from Schwann cells of the eighth cranial nerve

m. Fracture to one side of a structure caused by trauma to the other side

n. Fracture causing a portion of the skull to be pushed into the cranial cavity

o. Fracture of the zygomatic arch and orbital floor or rim and dislocation of the frontozygomatic suture

p. Malignant neoplasm of plasma cells involving the bone marrow and causing destruction of the bone

Exercise 6

Instructions: This exercise is a comprehensive review of the osteology and arthrology of the skull. Fill in missing words or provide a short answer for each item.

1. The bones of the skull are divided into two major groups, the _____ bones and the _____ bones.

2. List the cranial bones by name and quantity.

3. List the facial bones by name and quantity.

4. List the three classifications of fundamental skull shapes and indicate the number of degrees of angulation (formed by the petrous pyramids and the midsagittal plane) for each classification.

5. The bones of the cranial vault are classified as _____ bones.

6. The inner layer of spongy tissue found inside cranial bones is called _____.

7. The two fontanels located on the midsagittal plane of the skull are the _____ and the _____.

8. The fontanel located at the junction of the coronal and sagittal sutures is the _____.

9. The fontanel located at the junction of the lambdoidal and sagittal sutures is the _____.

10. The bone that forms the anterior portion of the cranium is the _____ bone.

11. The cranial bone located between the orbits and posterior to the nasal bones is the _____ bone.

12. The cranial bones that form the vertex and most of the sides of the cranium are the _____ bones.

13. The prominent bulge of a parietal bone is called the parietal _____.

14. The two parietal bones join together to form the _____ suture.

15. The two parietal bones articulate with the frontal bone to form the _____ suture.

16. The two parietal bones articulate posteriorly with the _____ bone.

17. The two parietal bones and the occipital bone join together to form the _____ suture.

18. The cranial bone that provides a depression to house the pituitary gland is the _____ bone.

19. The cranial bone that forms the posteroinferior portion of the cranium is the _____ bone.

20. The portion of the occipital bone that projects anteriorly from the foramen magnum is the _____ portion.

21. The large opening of the occipital bone through which part of the medulla oblongata passes is the

    _____ _____.

22. The basilar portion of the occipital bone fuses anteriorly

    with the body of the _____ bone.

23. The structure that articulates with the occipital condyles is

    the _____.

24. The middle portion of the cranial base is formed by the

    _____ bone.

25. The organs of hearing are located in the

    _____ bone.

26. The structure that separates the external acoustic meatus (EAM) from the auditory ossicles is the

    _____ membrane.

27. The process of the temporal bone that encloses radio-graphically significant air cells is the

    _____ process.

28. The thickest and densest portion of bone in the cranium is

    the _____ _____.

29. The petrous portion is a part of the

    _____ bone.

30. The fibrocartilaginous, oval-shaped portion of the external

    ear is the _____.

31. The three auditory ossicles are the _____,

    the _____, and the _____.

32. The zygomatic process projects anteriorly from the

    _____ bone.

33. The bone that forms part of the cranial base between the greater wings of the sphenoid bone and the occipital bone

    is the _____ bone.

34. The facial bones that form the bridge of the nose are the

    _____ bones.

35. The anterior portion of the medial walls of the orbits is

    formed by the _____ bones.

36. The largest of the immovable bones of the face is the

    _____ bone.

37. The body of each maxilla contains a large, pyramidal cavity called the _____

    _____.

38. The thick ridge on the inferior border of the maxillary bone

    that supports the teeth is the _____

    _____.

39. The anterior nasal spine projects superiorly from the

    _____.

40. The radiographically significant landmark that is the mid-point of the anterior nasal spine is the

    _____.

41. The facial bones that form the inferolateral portion of the

    orbital margin are the _____ bones.

42. The facial bones that form the prominence of the cheeks

    are the _____ bones.

43. The facial bones that form the posterior one fourth of the

    roof of the mouth are the _____ bones.

44. The scroll-like bony tissues that extend along the lateral

    walls of the nasal cavity are the _____

    _____ _____.

45. The facial bone forming the inferior part of the nasal sep-

    tum is the _____.

46. The largest and densest bone of the face is the

    _____.

47. The portion of the mandible that extends superiorly from the posterior aspect of the mandibular body is the

    _____.

48. The U-shaped bone located at the base of the tongue is the

    _____ bone.

49. The two processes that extend superiorly from a mandibular ramus are the _____ and the

    _____ process.

50. The part of the mandible that articulates with the mandibular fossa of the temporal bone to form the temporomandibular joint is the _____.

SECTION 2

Radiography of the Skull

Exercise 1: Skull Topography

Instructions: This exercise pertains to positioning landmarks used in skull radiography. Identify landmarks or provide a short answer for each item.

1. Identify each lettered positioning landmark shown in Fig. 20-14.

   A. _____

   B. _____

   C. _____

   D. _____

   E. _____

   F. _____

   G. _____

   H. _____

   I. _____

   J. _____

2. Identify each lettered positioning landmark shown in Fig. 20-15.

   A. _____

   B. _____

   C. _____

   D. _____

   E. _____

   F. _____

   G. _____

   H. _____

   I. _____

   J. _____

   K. _____

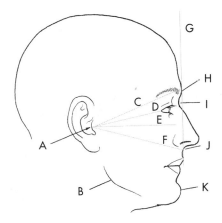

Figure 20-15 Lateral aspect landmarks.

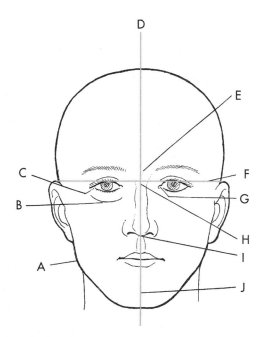

Figure 20-14 Anterior aspect landmarks.

3. Match the definitions in Column A with the appropriate term from Column B. Each term may be used only once.

Column A

_____ 1.   Midpoint of the frontonasal suture

_____ 2.   Midpoint of the anterior nasal spine

_____ 3.   Posterior surface of the occipital bone

_____ 4.   Smooth elevation between the superciliary arches

_____ 5.   Lateral aspect of each orbit; where the two eyelids originate

_____ 6.   Angle of the mandible; lateroposterior aspect of the mandible

_____ 7.   Superior aspect of the cranium; where the parietal bones join together

_____ 8.   Raised prominence just above each orbit on the frontal bone; coincides with the eyebrows

_____ 9.   Midpoint of the mental protuberance; anterior aspect of the mandible; where the two mandibular bodies join together

Column B

a. Inion

b. Vertex

c. Nasion

d. Gonion

e. Glabella

f. Acanthion

g. Mental point

h. Outer canthus

i. Superciliary arch

4. Match the definitions in Column A with the appropriate terms in Column B. The terms represent skull topography lines or planes. Each term may be used once, more than once, or not at all.

Column A

_____ 1.   Line extending across the front through both eyes

_____ 2.   Plane dividing the skull into equal right and left halves

_____ 3.   Line extending from the glabella to the anterior aspect of the maxilla

_____ 4.   Line extending from the EAM to the outer canthus

_____ 5.   Line extending from the EAM to the inferior margin of the orbit

_____ 6.   Line extending from the EAM to the midpoint of the anterior nasal spine

_____ 7.   Line extending from the EAM to the smooth elevation between the superciliary arches

Column B

a. Sagittal

b. Midsagittal

c. Midcoronal

d. Orbitomeatal

e. Interpupillary

f. Glabellomeatal

g. Acanthiomeatal

h. Glabelloalveolar

i. Infraorbitomeatal

5. How many degrees exist in the angles formed by the following lines?

   a. Orbitomeatal and infraorbitomeatal lines: _____

   b. Orbitomeatal and glabellomeatal lines: _____

Exercise 2: Positioning for the Cranium

Instructions: The typical radiographic evaluation of the skull, usually referred to as a skull series, involves a series of radiographs that may include a posteroanterior (PA) or anteroposterior (AP) projection, an AP axial projection, a full basal view, and one or two lateral views. This exercise pertains to those projections. Identify structures, fill in missing words, provide a short answer, select from a list, or choose true or false (explaining any statement you believe to be false) for each item.

Items 1 through 12 pertain to the *lateral projection*. Examine Fig. 20-16 as you answer the following items.

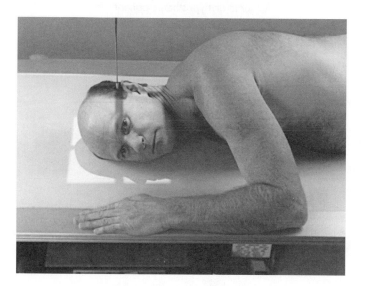

Figure 20-16 Lateral skull.

1. Which size image receptor (IR) should be used for average-sized adult skulls, and how should it be placed in the IR holder?

   a. 18 × 24 cm; crosswise
   b. 18 × 24 cm; lengthwise
   c. 24 × 30 cm; crosswise
   d. 24 × 30 cm; lengthwise

2. Indicate how the midsagittal plane and the interpupillary line should be positioned—perpendicular or parallel—with reference to the plane of the image receptor.

   a. Midsagittal plane: _____

   b. Interpupillary line: _____

3. Which positioning line of the head should be parallel with the plane of the image receptor?

   a. Interpupillary line
   b. Glabelloalveolar line
   c. Infraorbitomeatal line (IOML)

4. Which structure should be nearest to the center of the midline of the grid?

   a. Acanthion
   b. Zygoma bone
   c. Outer canthus
   d. External acoustic meatus

5. To what level of the patient should the IR be centered?

6. Describe how and where the central ray should be directed.

7. For cross-table lateral projections with the patient supine, which procedure should be performed to ensure that the entire cranium is included in the image?

   a. Elevate the head on a radiolucent sponge.
   b. Increase the source-to-image receptor distance (SID) to 72 inches.
   c. Use an 18 × 24 cm image receptor positioned lengthwise relative to the skull.

8. True or False. For cross-table lateral projections with the patient supine, the central ray should enter the side of the head at a point 2 inches (5 cm) anterior to the external acoustic meatus.

9. True or False. For cross-table lateral projections with the patient supine, a vertically oriented grid IR should be placed against the side of interest.

10. From the following list, circle the eight evaluation criteria that indicate the patient was properly positioned for a lateral projection.

    a. The petrous ridges should be symmetric.

    b. The sella turcica should be seen in profile.

    c. The orbital roofs should be superimposed.

    d. The mastoid regions should be superimposed.

    e. The mandible should not overlap the cervical vertebrae.

    f. The greater wings of sphenoid should be superimposed.

    g. The temporomandibular joints should be superimposed.

    h. The external acoustic meatuses should be superimposed.

    i. The dorsum sellae should be within the foramen magnum.

    j. The entire cranium should be demonstrated without rotation or tilt.

    k. The mental protuberance should be superimposed over the anterior frontal bone.

    l. The distance from the lateral border of the skull to the lateral border of the orbit should be equal on both sides.

11. Fig. 20-17 shows two diagrams of a recumbent patient with the midsagittal plane improperly aligned. Examine the diagrams and explain how the position of the patient in each should be adjusted to properly align the midsagittal plane with the image receptor.

    a. Diagram A:

    b. Diagram B:

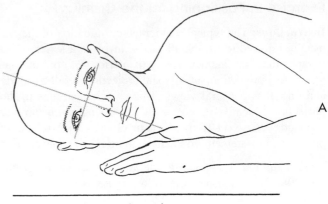

Asthenic or hyposthenic patient

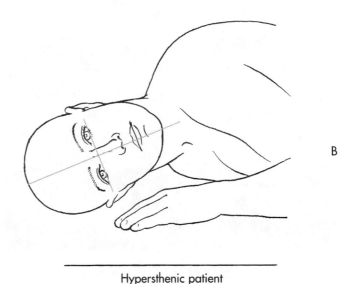

Hypersthenic patient

Figure 20-17 Adjusting the midsagittal plane with the patient in the recumbent position: **A,** Asthenic or hyposthenic patient. **B,** Hypersthenic patient.

12. Identify each lettered structure shown in Fig. 20-18.

   A. _____

   B. _____

   C. _____

   D. _____

   E. _____

   F. _____

   G. _____

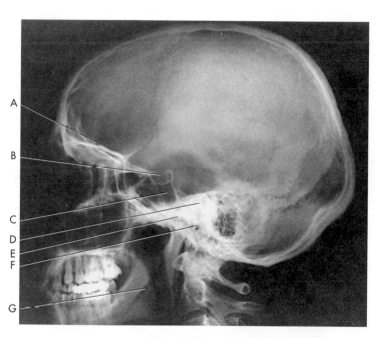

Figure 20-18 Lateral skull.

Items 13 through 20 pertain to *PA and PA axial projections.* Examine Figs. 20-19 and 20-20 as you answer the following items.

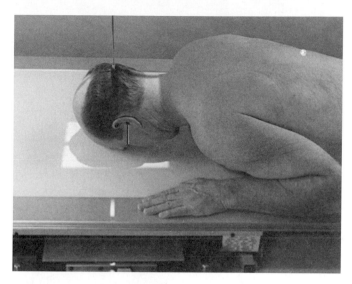

Figure 20-19 PA skull.

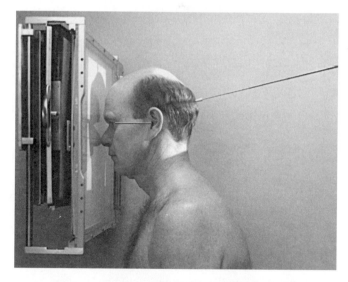

Figure 20-20 PA axial skull.

13. Indicate how the midsagittal plane and the orbitomeatal line (OML) should be positioned—perpendicular or parallel—with reference to the plane of the image receptor.

   a. Midsagittal plane: _____

   b. Orbitomeatal line: _____

14. Which parts of the patient's facial area should be in contact with the table or vertical grid device?
   a. Chin and nose
   b. Chin and cheek
   c. Forehead and nose
   d. Forehead and cheek

15. To demonstrate each of the following structures (Column A), identify how the central ray should be directed (Column B) with the patient positioned for a PA projection of the skull.

Column A

_____ 1. Frontal bone

_____ 2. General survey

_____ 3. Rotundum foramina

_____ 4. Superior orbital fissures

Column B

a. Perpendicular

b. 15 degrees caudad

c. 20 to 25 degrees caudad

d. 25 to 30 degrees caudad

16. The central ray should exit the skull at the

_____.

17. The IR should be centered to the skull at the level of the

_____.

18. What breathing instructions should be given to the patient?

19. From the following list, circle the five evaluation criteria that indicate the patient was properly positioned for either PA or PA axial projections.

a. The petrous ridges should be symmetric.
b. The orbital roofs should be superimposed.
c. The entire cranial perimeter should be included.
d. The mandible should not overlap the cervical vertebrae.
e. The dorsum sellae should be within the foramen magnum.
f. The mental protuberance should be superimposed over the anterior frontal bone.
g. The frontal bone should be penetrated without excessive density at the lateral borders of the skull.
h. The distance from the lateral border of the skull to the lateral border of the orbit should be equal on both sides.
i. The petrous pyramids should lie in the lower one third of the orbit with a central ray angulation of 15 degrees caudad and should fill the orbits with no central ray angulation.

20. Identify each lettered structure shown in Fig. 20-21.

A. _____

B. _____

C. _____

D. _____

E. _____

F. _____

G. _____

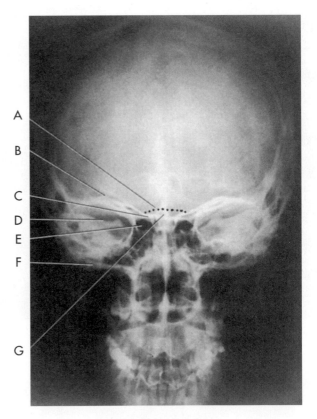

Figure 20-21 PA skull.

Items 21 through 27 pertain to *AP and AP axial projections.* Examine Figs. 20-22 and 20-23 as you answer the following items.

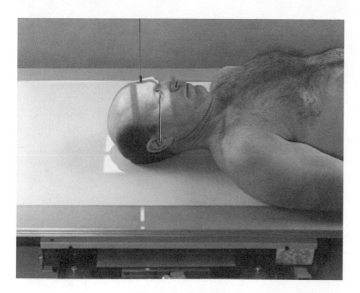

Figure 20-22 AP skull.

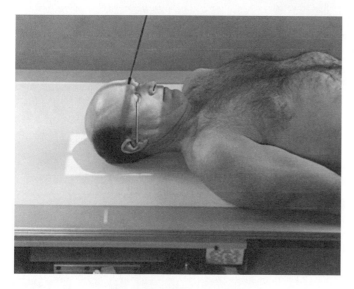

Figure 20-23 AP axial skull.

21. Indicate how the midsagittal plane and the orbitomeatal line should be positioned—perpendicular or parallel—with reference to the plane of the image receptor.

   a. Midsagittal plane: _____

   b. Orbitomeatal line: _____

22. For the AP projection, the central ray should be directed _____ (caudally, cephalically, or perpendicularly).

23. For the AP axial projection, the central ray should be directed _____ (caudally, cephalically, or perpendicularly).

24. When performing either the AP or AP axial projection for general surveys of the skull, where on the skull should the central ray be directed?
   a. Nasion
   b. Acanthion
   c. Tip of the nose

25. Which of the following image characteristics indicates that a general survey image of the skull is an AP projection instead of a PA projection?
   a. The petrous ridges are symmetric.
   b. The petrous pyramids fill the orbits.
   c. The orbits are considerably magnified.
   d. The entire cranial perimeter is demonstrated.

26. From the following list, circle the five evaluation criteria that indicate the patient was properly positioned for either the AP or AP axial projections.
   a. The petrous ridges should be symmetric.
   b. The orbital roofs should be superimposed.
   c. The entire cranial perimeter should be included.
   d. The mandible should not overlap the cervical vertebrae.
   e. The dorsum sellae should be within the foramen magnum.
   f. The mental protuberance should be superimposed over the anterior frontal bone.
   g. The frontal bone should be penetrated without excessive density at the lateral borders of the skull.
   h. The distance from the lateral border of the skull to the lateral border of the orbit should be equal on both sides.
   i. The petrous pyramids should lie in the lower one third of the orbit, with a central ray angulation of 15 degrees caudad, and should fill the orbits with no central ray angulation.
   j. The petrous pyramids should lie in the lower one third of the orbit, with a central ray angulation of 15 degrees cephalically, and should fill the orbits with no central ray angulation.

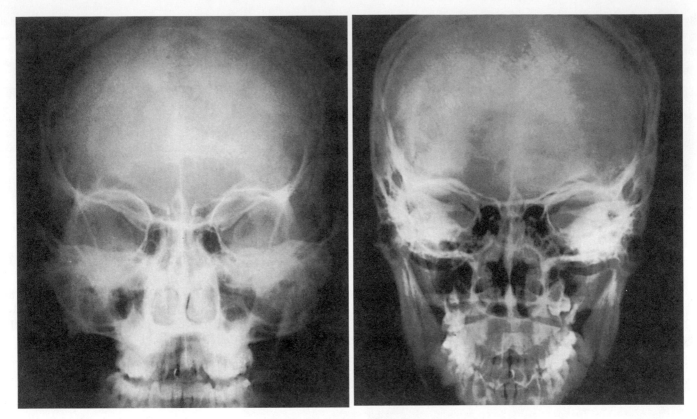

Figure 20-24 Two views of the skull.

27. Fig. 20-24 shows two skull radiographs: one AP and one AP axial. Examine each image and state how the central ray was directed by indicating how specific structures appear in relation to the surrounding structures.

a. Diagram A:

_____

_____

_____

b. Diagram B:

_____

_____

_____

Items 28 through 35 pertain to the *AP axial projection, Towne method.* Examine Fig. 20-25 as you answer the following items.

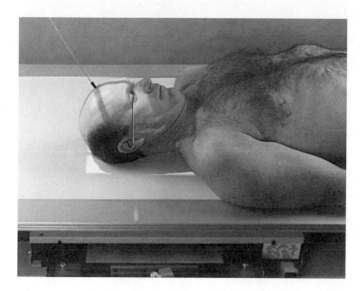

Figure 20-25 AP axial skull, Towne method.

28. Which size IR should be used for average-sized adult skulls, and how should it be placed in the IR holder?

   a. 18 × 24 cm; crosswise
   b. 18 × 24 cm; lengthwise
   c. 24 × 30 cm; crosswise
   d. 24 × 30 cm; lengthwise

29. To what level of the patient should the upper border of the IR be aligned?

   a. Nasion
   b. Glabella
   c. Highest point of the vertex

30. In addition to the midsagittal plane, either the

   _____ line or the

   _____ line must be perpendicular to the plane of the image receptor.

31. Which two central ray angulations could be used to properly perform the AP axial projection?

   a. 30 degrees caudad and 37 degrees caudad
   b. 30 degrees caudad and 37 degrees cephalad
   c. 30 degrees cephalad and 37 degrees caudad
   d. 30 degrees cephalad and 37 degrees cephalad

32. Which positioning factor determines the number of degrees that the central ray should be angled?

   a. The type of skull being positioned
   b. Whether the patient is supine or seated upright
   c. How much source-to-image receptor distance is used
   d. Which positioning line is perpendicular to the image receptor

33. Where exactly on the patient's head should the central ray enter?

   a. 1 inch (2.5 cm) above the nasion
   b. 1 inch (2.5 cm) below the nasion
   c. 2 to 2½ inches (5 to 6.25 cm) above the glabella
   d. 2 to 2½ inches (5 to 6.25 cm) below the glabella

34. From the following list, circle the four evaluation criteria that indicate the patient was properly positioned for the AP axial projection, Towne method.

   a. The orbital roofs should be superimposed.
   b. The petrous pyramids should be symmetric.
   c. The mandible should not overlap the cervical vertebrae.
   d. The petrous pyramids should lie in the lower one third of the orbits.
   e. The mental protuberance should be superimposed over the anterior frontal bone.
   f. The occipital bone should be penetrated without excessive density at the lateral borders of the skull.
   g. The dorsum sellae and posterior clinoid processes should be visualized within the foramen magnum.
   h. The distance from the lateral border of the skull to the lateral border of the orbit should be equal on both sides.
   i. The distance from the lateral border of the skull to the lateral margin of the foramen magnum should be equal on both sides.

35. Identify each lettered structure shown in Fig. 20-26.

A. _____

B. _____

C. _____

D. _____

E. _____

F. _____

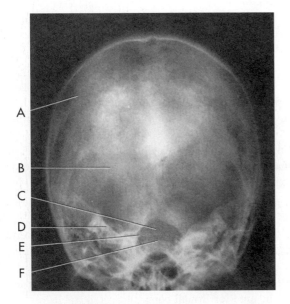

Figure 20-26 AP axial skull, Towne method.

Items 36 through 43 pertain to the *PA axial projection, Haas method*. Examine Fig. 20-27 as you answer the following items.

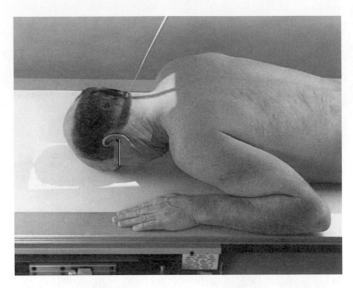

Figure 20-27 PA axial skull, Haas method.

36. True or False. The PA axial projection, Haas method, demonstrates the occipital region of the cranium.

37. True or False. Hypersthenic patients should be positioned while recumbent in the supine position.

38. Which parts of the patient's head should be in contact with the table or vertical grid device?

a. Chin and nose
b. Chin and cheek
c. Forehead and nose
d. Forehead and cheek

39. In addition to the midsagittal plane, which positioning line of the skull should be perpendicular to the plane of the image receptor?

a. Orbitomeatal
b. Glabellomeatal
c. Acanthiomeatal
d. Infraorbitomeatal

40. How many degrees and in which direction should the central ray be directed?

    a. 25 degrees caudad
    b. 25 degrees cephalad
    c. 30 degrees caudad
    d. 30 degrees cephalad

41. Where on the midsagittal plane of the patient's skull should the central ray enter?

    a. At the vertex of the skull
    b. At a point approximately $1^1/_2$ inches (3.8 cm) above the external occipital protuberance
    c. At a point approximately $1^1/_2$ inches (3.8 cm) below the external occipital protuberance
    d. At a point approximately 3 inches (7.6 cm) below the external occipital protuberance

42. From the following list, circle the four evaluation criteria that indicate the patient was properly positioned for the PA axial projection, Haas method.

    a. The entire cranium should be included.
    b. The orbital roofs should be superimposed.
    c. The petrous pyramids should be symmetric.
    d. The mandible should not overlap the cervical vertebrae.
    e. The petrous pyramids should lie in the lower one third of the orbits.
    f. The mental protuberance should be superimposed over the anterior frontal bone.
    g. The dorsum sellae and posterior clinoid processes should be seen within the foramen magnum.
    h. The distance from the lateral border of the skull to the lateral border of the orbit should be equal on both sides.
    i. The distance from the lateral border of the skull to the lateral border of the foramen magnum should be equal on both sides.

43. Identify each lettered structure shown in Fig. 20-28.

    A. _____

    B. _____

    C. _____

    D. _____

    E. _____

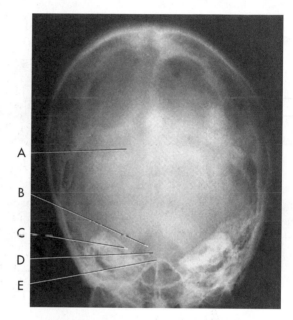

Figure 20-28 PA axial skull, Haas method.

Items 44 through 50 pertain to the *submentovertical (SMV) projection, Schüller method.* Examine Fig. 20-29 as you answer the following items.

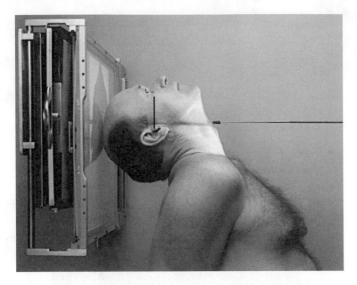

Figure 20-29 SMV cranial base.

44. Indicate how the midsagittal plane and the infraorbitomeatal line should be positioned—perpendicular or parallel—with reference to the plane of the image receptor.

   a. Midsagittal plane: _____

   b. Infraorbitomeatal: _____

45. To what positioning line of the skull should the perpendicular central ray be directed?

   _____

46. Describe where the central ray should enter the patient.

47. Through which cranial structure should the central ray pass?

   a. Sella turcica
   b. Ethmoidal air cells
   c. External acoustic meatus

48. From the following list, select the two positioning factors on which the success of submentovertical projections most depend.

   a. Directing the central ray perpendicular to the OML
   b. Directing the central ray perpendicular to the IOML
   c. Directing the central ray perpendicular to the midsagittal plane
   d. Placing the OML as near as possible to parallel with the plane of the image receptor
   e. Placing the IOML as near as possible to parallel with the plane of the image receptor
   f. Placing the midsagittal plane as near as possible to parallel with the plane of the image receptor

49. From the following list, circle the five evaluation criteria that indicate the patient was properly positioned for a SMV projection.

   a. The petrosae should be symmetric.
   b. The orbital roofs should be superimposed.
   c. The mandibular rami should be superimposed.
   d. The mental protuberance should superimpose the anterior frontal bone.
   e. The petrous pyramids should lie in the lower one third of the orbits.
   f. The mandibular condyles should be anterior to the petrous pyramids.
   g. The dorsum sellae should be seen and projected within the foramen magnum.
   h. The structures of the cranial base should be clearly visible as indicated by adequate penetration.
   i. The distance from the lateral border of the skull to the mandibular condyles should be equal on both sides.

50. Identify each lettered structure shown in Fig. 20-30.

A. _____   F. _____

B. _____   G. _____

C. _____   H. _____

D. _____   I. _____

E. _____

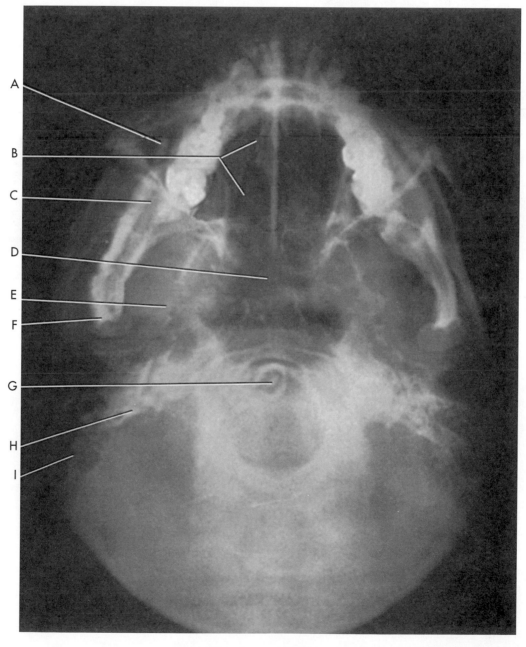

Figure 20-30 SMV cranial base.

Items 51 through 55 pertain to the *verticosubmental (VSM) projection, Schüller method.* Examine Fig. 20-31 as you answer the following items.

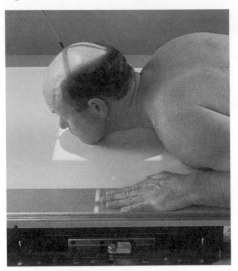

Figure 20-31 VSM cranial base.

51. The verticosubmental projection is often performed in place of which of the following projections?

   a. AP axial, Towne method
   b. PA axial, Caldwell method
   c. Submentovertical, Schüller method

52. Into which body position should the patient be placed?

   a. Prone
   b. Supine
   c. Upright
   d. Lateral recumbent

53. Which part of the patient's head should be placed on the table?

   a. Ear
   b. Chin
   c. Vertex
   d. Forehead

54. From the following list, select three characteristics concerning how the central ray should be directed.

   a. Perpendicular to the OML
   b. Perpendicular to the IOML
   c. Directed to exit at the glabella
   d. Directed to exit at the acanthion
   e. Directed through the sella turcica
   f. Directed to the external occipital protuberance
   g. Perpendicular to the center of the image receptor
   h. Passes through a point $^3/_4$ inch (1.9 cm) anterior to the level of the EAMs

55. Identify each lettered structure shown in Fig. 20-32.

A. _____

B. _____

C. _____

D. _____

E. _____

F. _____

G. _____

H. _____

I. _____

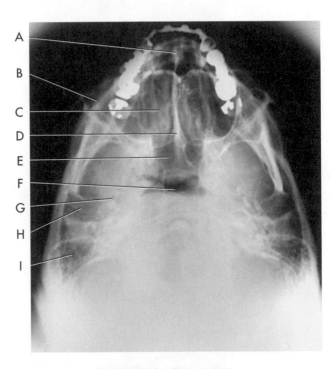

Figure 20-32 VSM cranial base.

Exercise 3: Positioning for the Sella Turcica

Instructions: To supplement computed tomography, a tightly collimated image of the sella turcica is often requested. This exercise pertains to the lateral projection of the sella turcica. Provide a short answer, select from a list, or identify structures for each item.

Examine Fig. 20-33 as you answer the following items about the *lateral projection for the sella turcica.*

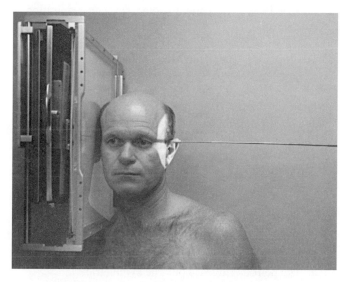

Figure 20-33 Lateral skull for the sella turcica.

1. Indicate how each of the following should be adjusted—perpendicular or parallel—to correctly position the patient for lateral projections of the sella turcica.

   a. Midsagittal plane: _____

   b. Interpupillary line: _____

   c. Infraorbitomeatal line: _____

2. Where exactly on the side of the head should the central ray enter?

3. What breathing instructions should be given to the patient?

4. From the following list, circle the four evaluation criteria that indicate the patient was properly positioned for a lateral projection of the sella turcica.

   a. The sella turcica should not be rotated or distorted.
   b. The anterior clinoid processes should be superimposed.
   c. The posterior clinoid processes should be superimposed.
   d. The sella turcica should be in the center of the radiograph.
   e. The petrous pyramids should lie in the lower one third of the orbits.
   f. The dorsum sellae should be seen and projected within the foramen magnum.
   g. The distance from the lateral border of the skull to the mandibular condyles should be equal on both sides.

5. Identify each lettered structure shown in Fig. 20-34.

   A. _____

   B. _____

   C. _____

   D. _____

   E. _____

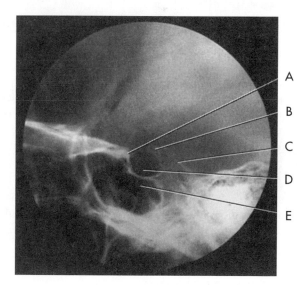

Figure 20-34 Lateral sella turcica.

Exercise 4: Positioning for the Optic Canal and Foramen

Instructions: Parietoorbital oblique projections and orbitoparietal oblique projections are two standard radiographic procedures used to demonstrate the orbital region, specifically the optic canal and foramen. This exercise pertains to those types of projections. Identify structures, select from a list, provide a short answer, or choose true or false (explaining any statement you believe to be false) for each item.

Items 1 through 10 pertain to the *parietoorbital oblique projection, Rhese method.* Examine Fig. 20-35 as you answer the following items.

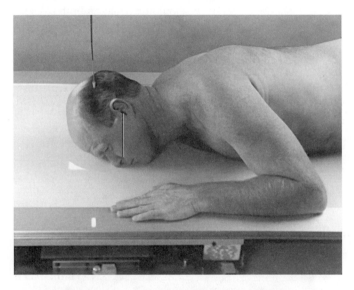

Figure 20-35 Parietoorbital oblique projection, Rhese method.

1. In addition to the zygoma and nose, which other structure should be in contact with the x-ray table or vertical grid device?

   a. Ear
   b. Chin
   c. Forehead

2. Which positioning line of the head should be perpendicular to the plane of the image receptor?

   a. Interpupillary
   b. Acanthiomeatal
   c. Infraorbitomeatal

3. Which body plane or positioning line should form an angle of 53 degrees with the plane of the image receptor?

   a. Midsagittal plane
   b. Midcoronal plane
   c. Interpupillary line
   d. Acanthiomeatal line

4. True or False. Of the two orbits, the affected orbit should be placed closest to the image receptor.

5. True or False. The patient should suspend respiration for the exposure.

6. True or False. The central ray should be directed caudally 15 degrees.

7. True or False. The parietoorbital oblique projection demonstrates a cross-sectional view of the optic canal.

8. True or False. Incorrect angulation of the acanthiomeatal line will cause lateral deviation from the preferred location of the optic canal in the imaged orbit.

9. From the following list, circle the four evaluation criteria that indicate the patient was properly positioned for a parietoorbital oblique projection.

   a. The petrous ridges should be symmetric.
   b. The entire orbital rim should be included.
   c. The orbital roofs should be superimposed.
   d. The dorsum sellae should be within the foramen magnum.
   e. The supraorbital margins should lie in the same horizontal line.
   f. The optic canal and foramen should be seen at the end of the sphenoid ridge.
   g. The optic canal and foramen should lie in the inferior and lateral quadrant of the orbit.
   h. The optic canal and foramen should lie in the superior and medial quadrant of the orbit.

10. Identify each lettered structure shown in Fig. 20-36.

A. _____

B. _____

C. _____

D. _____

E. _____

F. _____

G. _____

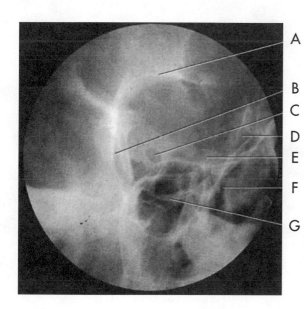

Figure 20-36 Parietoorbital oblique projection.

Items 11 through 20 pertain to the *orbitoparietal oblique projection, Rhese method.* Examine Fig. 20-37 as you answer the following items.

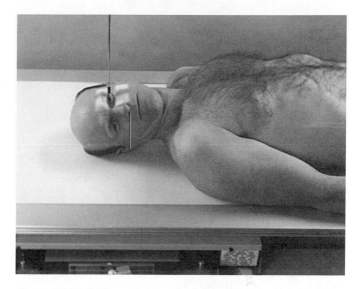

Figure 20-37 Orbitoparietal oblique projection, Rhese method.

11. True or False. The patient should be positioned from either the seated (upright) position or the supine position.

12. True or False. Of the two orbits, the affected orbit should be placed farthest from the image receptor.

13. True or False. The central ray should enter the affected orbit.

14. True or False. The orbitoparietal oblique projection causes less radiation exposure to the lens of the eye than the parietoorbital oblique projection.

15. True or False. The orbitoparietal oblique projection results in more magnification of the orbit than the parietoorbital oblique projection.

16. What positioning line of the head should be perpendicular to the image receptor?

17. What plane of the body should form an angle of 53 degrees with the image receptor?

18. How should the central ray be directed?

    a. Perpendicularly
    b. 53 degrees caudally
    c. 53 degrees cephalically

19. Which projection produces an image similar to that of the orbitoparietal oblique projection?

    a. Submentovertical projection
    b. Parietoorbital oblique projection
    c. PA axial projection, Haas method

20. From the following list, circle the four evaluation criteria that indicate the patient was properly positioned for an orbitoparietal oblique projection.

    a. The petrous ridges should be symmetric.
    b. The orbital roofs should be superimposed.
    c. The entire orbital rim should be included.
    d. The dorsum sellae should be within the foramen magnum.
    e. The supraorbital margins should lie in the same horizontal line.
    f. The optic canal and foramen should be seen at the end of the sphenoid ridge.
    g. The optic canal and foramen should lie in the inferior and lateral quadrant of the orbit.
    h. The optic canal and foramen should lie in the superior and medial quadrant of the orbit.

Exercise 5: Evaluating Radiographs of the Skull

Instructions: This exercise consists of radiographs of the skull, most of which show at least one positioning error, to give you some practice evaluating skull positioning. These images are not from *Merrill's Atlas of Radiographic Positions and Radiologic Procedures*. Examine each image and answer the questions that follow by providing a short answer.

1. Figs. 20-38 through 20-40 are lateral projection radiographs of a phantom skull. Only one image demonstrates acceptable positioning. Examine the images and answer the questions that follow. Refer to specific evaluation criteria for this projection when explaining your answers.

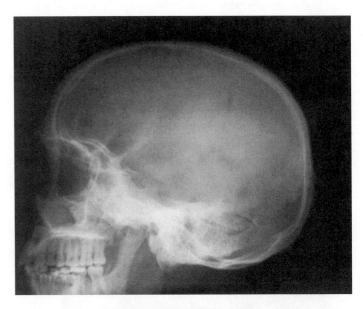

Figure 20-38 Lateral skull.

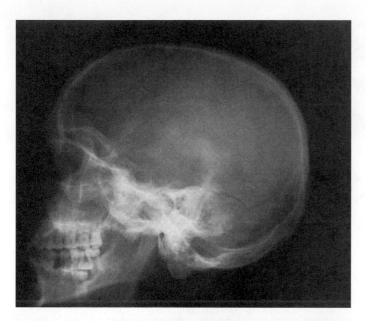

Figure 20-39 Lateral skull.

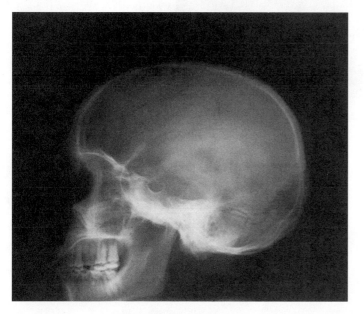

Figure 20-40 Lateral skull.

a. Which image best demonstrates an optimally positioned skull? Explain.

b. Which image shows the skull incorrectly positioned because the vertex and midsagittal plane are tilted toward the plane of the image receptor? Explain.

c. Which image shows the skull incorrectly positioned because the face and midsagittal plane are rotated toward the x-ray table and image receptor? Explain.

d. Which image shows the skull positioned similarly to that seen in Fig. 20-17, Diagram B?

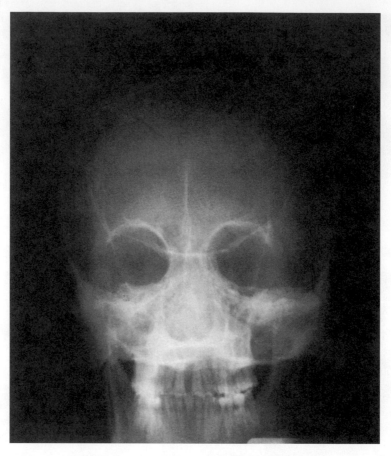

Figure 20-41 PA skull showing incorrect positioning.

2. Fig. 20-41 shows a PA projection radiograph of a phantom skull with incorrect positioning. Examine the image and answer the questions that follow.

a. Assuming that the OML was perpendicular to the plane of the IR, describe how the central ray most likely was directed.

c. What image characteristic most likely prevents this image from meeting all the evaluation criteria for this projection?

b. Describe where the petrous ridges should appear in the image when the central ray is directed caudally 15 degrees.

d. Describe the positioning error that most likely caused the image to appear as it does.

3. Fig. 20-42 shows a PA projection radiograph of a phantom skull with incorrect positioning. Examine the image and answer the questions that follow.

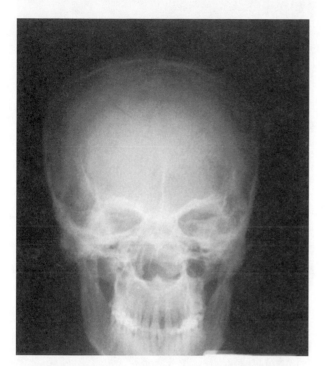

Figure 20-42 PA skull showing incorrect positioning.

a. Assuming that the OML was perpendicular to the plane of the IR, describe how the central ray most likely was directed.

b. Describe where the petrous ridges should appear in the image when the central ray is directed caudally 15 degrees.

c. Do the petrous ridges nearly fill the orbits?

d. What image characteristic most likely prevents this image from meeting all evaluation criteria for this projection?

e. Describe the positioning error that most likely caused the image to appear as it does.

4. Figs. 20-43 and 20-44 show AP projection radiographs of a phantom skull. Only one image demonstrates acceptable positioning. Examine the images and answer the questions that follow.

   a. Is the positioning quality for Fig. 20-43 acceptable or unacceptable?

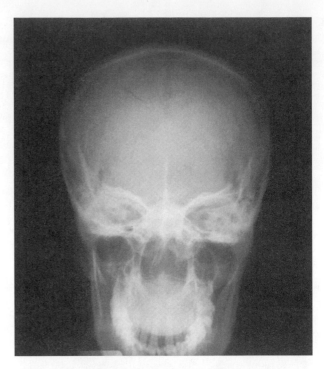

Figure 20-43 AP projection.

   b. Is the positioning quality for Fig. 20-44 acceptable or unacceptable?

   c. Describe the positioning error that probably caused the unacceptable image.

   d. Assuming that the OML was perpendicular for both images, in which way does the central ray appear to have been directed?

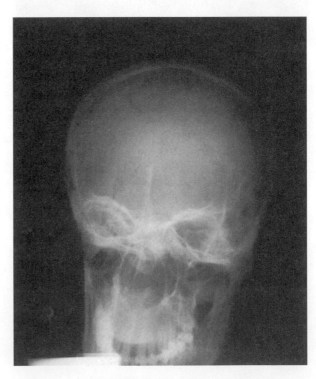

Figure 20-44 AP projection.

5. Examine Fig. 20-45 and state why it does not meet the evaluation criteria for this type of projection.

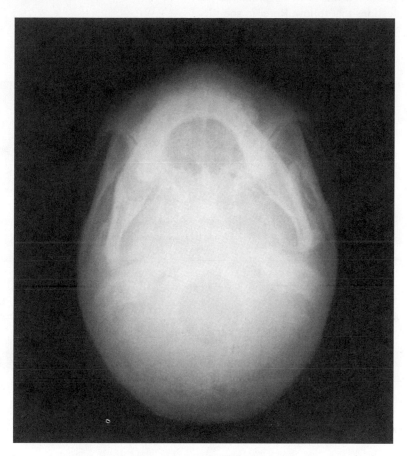

Figure 20-45 SMV projection showing incorrect positioning.

6. Figs. 20-46 through 20-48 are parietoorbital oblique projection radiographs of a phantom skull. Only one image demonstrates the correct rotation of the head. Examine the images and answer the questions that follow. Refer to specific evaluation criteria for this projection when explaining your answers.

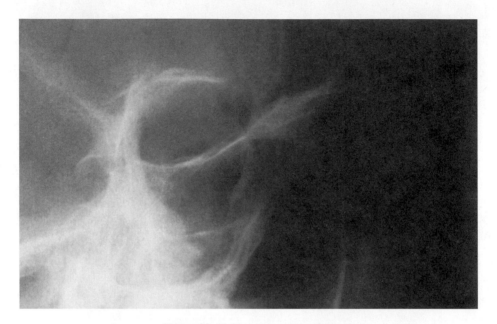

Figure 20-46 Phantom skull orbit.

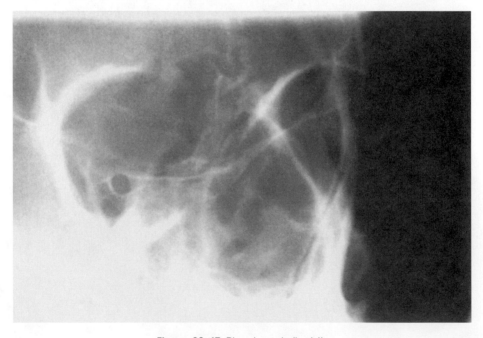

Figure 20-47 Phantom skull orbit.

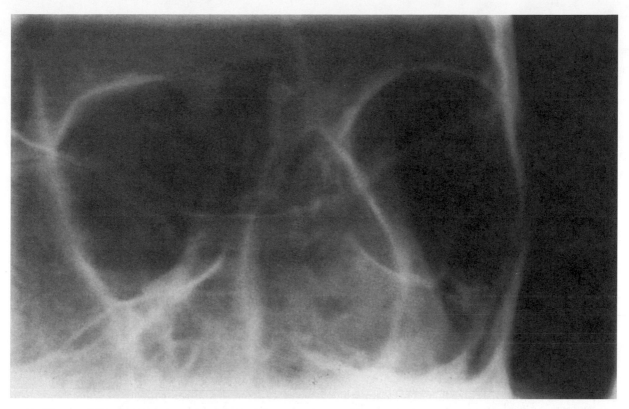

Figure 20-48 Phantom skull orbit.

a. Which image best demonstrates ideal positioning of the phantom skull? Explain.

b. In which image does the midsagittal plane form an angle with the IR that is considerably less than the required amount? Explain.

c. In which image does the midsagittal plane form an angle with the IR that is somewhat greater than the required amount? Explain.

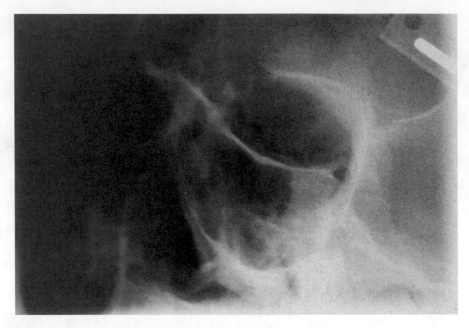

Figure 20-49 Orbitoparietal oblique projection showing incorrect positioning of a phantom skull.

7. Fig. 20-49 is an orbitoparietal oblique projection radiograph of the left orbit of a phantom skull that is incorrectly aligned. Examine the image and answer the questions that follow.

a. What image characteristic indicates that the phantom skull was not correctly positioned?

b. What positioning error most likely produced this image?

c. How should the patient's position be adjusted to improve the demonstration of orbital structures with a subsequent radiograph?

Note to Students: Additional exercises referenced from Chapters 20 through 23 are found in the Appendix (Supplemental Exercises for Skull Positioning), which is located in this workbook. Students should complete the review exercises for those chapters before completing the appendix exercises.

Self-Test: Osteology and Radiography of the Skull

Instructions: Answer the following questions by selecting the best choice.

1. Which positioning line extends from the EAM to the outer canthus?

   a. Orbitomeatal
   b. Glabellomeatal
   c. Acanthiomeatal
   d. Infraorbitomeatal

2. Which positioning landmark is located at the base of the nasal spine?

   a. Nasion
   b. Gonion
   c. Glabella
   d. Acanthion

3. Which positioning landmark is located at the most superior point of the nasal bones?

   a. Nasion
   b. Canthus
   c. Glabella
   d. Acanthion

4. Which positioning landmark is the smooth elevation that is located between the superciliary arches?

   a. Nasion
   b. Glabella
   c. Acanthion
   d. Mental point

5. Which positioning landmark is most superior?

   a. Nasion
   b. Gonion
   c. Glabella
   d. Acanthion

6. Where on the skull is the gonion located?

   a. Between the orbits
   b. On the anterior frontal bone
   c. On the posterior occipital bone
   d. On the lateroposterior part of the mandible

7. Where on the skull is the outer canthus located?

   a. Between the orbits
   b. At the mandibular angle
   c. Along each parietal eminence
   d. On the lateral border of each orbit

8. Which positioning landmark is located at the anterior portion of the mandible?

   a. Nasion
   b. Gonion
   c. Acanthion
   d. Mental point

9. Which suture articulates the frontal bone with both parietal bones?

   a. Sagittal
   b. Coronal
   c. Squamosal
   d. Lambdoidal

10. Which suture joins both parietal bones at the vertex of the skull?

    a. Sagittal
    b. Coronal
    c. Squamosal
    d. Lambdoidal

11. Which suture joins a parietal bone with both a sphenoid bone and a temporal bone?

    a. Sagittal
    b. Coronal
    c. Squamosal
    d. Lambdoidal

12. Which suture joins both parietal bones with the occipital bone?

    a. Sagittal
    b. Coronal
    c. Squamosal
    d. Lambdoidal

13. The bregma fontanel is located at the junction of which two sutures?

    a. Coronal and sagittal
    b. Coronal and squamosal
    c. Lambdoidal and sagittal
    d. Lambdoidal and squamosal

14. The lambda fontanel is located at the junction of which two sutures?

    a. Coronal and sagittal
    b. Coronal and squamosal
    c. Lambdoidal and sagittal
    d. Lambdoidal and squamosal

15. The bregma fontanel is located at the junction of which cranial bones?

    a. Frontal and both parietals
    b. Occipital and both parietals
    c. Frontal and sphenoid
    d. Occipital and sphenoid

16. The lambda fontanel is located at the junction of which cranial bones?

    a. Frontal and both parietals
    b. Occipital and both parietals
    c. Frontal and temporal
    d. Occipital and temporal

17. Which skull classification refers to a typical skull (in terms of width and length)?

    a. Mesocephalic
    b. Brachycephalic
    c. Dolichocephalic

18. Which skull classification refers to a long, narrow skull?
    a. Mesocephalic
    b. Brachycephalic
    c. Dolichocephalic

19. Which skull classification refers to a short, wide skull?

    a. Mesocephalic
    b. Brachycephalic
    c. Dolichocephalic

20. How many degrees are in the angle formed between the midsagittal plane and the petrous pyramids in the mesocephalic skull?

    a. 36 degrees
    b. 40 degrees
    c. 47 degrees
    d. 54 degrees

21. How many degrees are in the angle formed between the midsagittal plane and the petrous pyramids in the brachycephalic skull?

    a. 36 degrees
    b. 40 degrees
    c. 47 degrees
    d. 54 degrees

22. How many degrees are in the angle formed between the midsagittal plane and the petrous pyramids in the dolichocephalic skull?

    a. 36 degrees
    b. 40 degrees
    c. 47 degrees
    d. 54 degrees

23. On which cranial bone are the superciliary arches located?

    a. Frontal
    b. Parietal
    c. Ethmoid
    d. Occipital

24. On which cranial bone is the cribriform plate located?

    a. Frontal
    b. Ethmoid
    c. Temporal
    d. Sphenoid

25. On which cranial bone is the crista galli located?

    a. Ethmoid
    b. Occipital
    c. Temporal
    d. Sphenoid

26. Which cranial bone has a petrous pyramid?

    a. Parietal
    b. Ethmoid
    c. Temporal
    d. Sphenoid

27. On which cranial bone is the sella turcica located?

    a. Frontal
    b. Ethmoid
    c. Temporal
    d. Sphenoid

28. Which cranial bone has the mastoid process?

    a. Parietal
    b. Ethmoid
    c. Temporal
    d. Sphenoid

29. On which cranial bone is the perpendicular plate located?

    a. Parietal
    b. Ethmoid
    c. Temporal
    d. Sphenoid

30. Which cranial bone has both greater and lesser wings?

    a. Ethmoid
    b. Occipital
    c. Temporal
    d. Sphenoid

31. With which cranial bone does the first cervical vertebra articulate?

    a. Ethmoid
    b. Occipital
    c. Temporal
    d. Sphenoid

32. The pterygoid processes project inferiorly from which cranial bone?

    a. Frontal
    b. Ethmoid
    c. Temporal
    d. Sphenoid

33. The foramen magnum is a part of which cranial bone?

    a. Frontal
    b. Occipital
    c. Temporal
    d. Sphenoid

34. From which cranial bone does the zygomatic process arise?

    a. Frontal
    b. Parietal
    c. Temporal
    d. Sphenoid

35. The external acoustic meatus is a part of which cranial bone?

    a. Frontal
    b. Parietal
    c. Temporal
    d. Sphenoid

36. The temporal process projects posteriorly from which facial bone?

    a. Vomer
    b. Maxilla
    c. Zygoma
    d. Temporal

37. Which bones comprise the bridge of the nose?

    a. Nasal
    b. Lacrimal
    c. Palatine
    d. Maxillae

38. With which bone does the mandible articulate?

    a. Hyoid
    b. Maxilla
    c. Zygoma
    d. Temporal

39. Where are the lacrimal bones located?

    a. Inside the nasal cavity
    b. On the lateral wall of each orbit
    c. On the medial wall of each orbit
    d. Inferior to the maxillary sinuses

40. Where is the vomer bone found?

    a. Posterior to the nasal bones
    b. On the floor of the nasal cavity
    c. On the lateral wall of the orbits
    d. In the posterior one fourth of the roof of the mouth

41. Which bone comprises most of the lateral wall of the orbital cavities?

    a. Maxilla
    b. Lacrimal
    c. Palatine
    d. Zygomatic

42. Which term refers to the anterior process of the mandibular ramus?

    a. Cornu
    b. Condyle
    c. Coracoid
    d. Coronoid

43. Which term refers to the posterior process of the mandibular ramus?

    a. Cornu
    b. Condyle
    c. Coracoid
    d. Coronoid

44. Which facial bones have alveolar processes?

    a. Vomer and mandible
    b. Vomer and zygomatic
    c. Maxillae and mandible
    d. Maxillae and zygomatic

45. Which bones form the posterior one fourth of the roof of the mouth?

    a. Maxillae
    b. Palatine
    c. Zygomatic
    d. Inferior nasal conchae

46. Which positioning landmark is located on the maxillae?

    a. Gonion
    b. Nasion
    c. Acanthion
    d. Mental point

47. Which two positioning lines or planes should be perpendicular to the IR for the PA projection of the skull?

    a. Orbitomeatal line and midsagittal plane
    b. Orbitomeatal line and interpupillary line
    c. Infraorbitomeatal line and midsagittal plane
    d. Infraorbitomeatal line and interpupillary line

48. With reference to the patient, where should the IR be centered for the PA projection of the skull?

    a. Nasion
    b. Glabella
    c. Acanthion
    d. Mental point

49. With reference to the patient, where should the IR be centered for the lateral projection of the skull?

    a. Nasion
    b. External acoustic meatus
    c. 2 inches (5 cm) above the external acoustic meatus
    d. 2 inches (5 cm) below the external acoustic meatus

50. With reference to the IR, how should the interpupillary line and the midsagittal plane be positioned for the lateral projection of the skull?

    a. Interpupillary line: parallel; midsagittal plane: parallel
    b. Interpupillary line: parallel; midsagittal plane: perpendicular
    c. Interpupillary line: perpendicular; midsagittal plane: parallel
    d. Interpupillary line: perpendicular; midsagittal plane: perpendicular

51. For the AP axial projection, Towne method, of the skull, how many degrees and in which direction should the central ray be directed when the OML is perpendicular to the image receptor?

    a. 30 degrees caudad
    b. 30 degrees cephalad
    c. 37 degrees caudad
    d. 37 degrees cephalad

52. For the AP axial projection, Towne method, of the skull, how many degrees and in which direction should the central ray be directed when the IOML is perpendicular to the image receptor?

    a. 30 degrees caudad
    b. 30 degrees cephalad
    c. 37 degrees caudad
    d. 37 degrees cephalad

53. Which positioning line should be parallel with the IR for the SMV projection of the skull?

    a. Orbitomeatal line
    b. Glabellomeatal line
    c. Acanthiomeatal line
    d. Infraorbitomeatal line

54. Which projection of the skull can be correctly performed with the central ray angled 37 degrees?

    a. AP axial, Towne method
    b. PA axial, Haas method
    c. PA axial, Caldwell method
    d. Parietoorbital oblique, Rhese method

55. Which projection of the skull can be correctly performed with the central ray angled 15 degrees?

    a. Submentovertical
    b. AP axial, Towne method
    c. PA axial, Haas method
    d. PA axial, Caldwell method

56. Which projection of the skull produces a full basal image of the cranium?

    a. Lateral
    b. AP axial, Towne method
    c. PA with perpendicular central ray
    d. Submentovertical, Schüller method

57. Which projection of the skull projects the petrous bones in the lower third of the orbits?

    a. PA axial, Haas method
    b. AP axial, Towne method
    c. PA axial, Caldwell method
    d. PA with perpendicular central ray

58. Which projection of the skull should be obtained when the frontal bone is of primary interest?

    a. PA axial, Haas method
    b. AP axial, Towne method
    c. PA axial, Caldwell method
    d. PA with perpendicular central ray

59. Which evaluation criterion pertains to the AP axial projection, Towne method, of the skull?

    a. The orbital roofs should be superimposed.
    b. The mental protuberance should superimpose the anterior frontal bone.
    c. Part of the sella turcica should be seen within the foramen magnum.
    d. The distance from the lateral border of the skull to the lateral border of the orbit should be the same on both sides.

60. Which evaluation criterion pertains to the PA projection of the skull?
    a. The orbital roofs should be superimposed.
    b. The mental protuberance should superimpose the anterior frontal bone.
    c. Part of the sella turcica should be seen within the foramen magnum.
    d. The distance from the lateral border of the skull to the lateral border of the orbit should be the same on both sides.

61. Which evaluation criterion pertains to the lateral projection of the skull?
    a. The orbital roofs should be superimposed.
    b. The mental protuberance should superimpose the anterior frontal bone.
    c. Part of the sella turcica should be seen within the foramen magnum.
    d. The distance from the lateral border of the skull to the lateral border of the orbit should be the same on both sides.

62. Which evaluation criterion pertains to the SMV projection of the skull?
    a. The orbital roofs should be superimposed.
    b. The mental protuberance should superimpose the anterior frontal bone.
    c. Part of the sella turcica should be seen within the foramen magnum.
    d. The distance from the lateral border of the skull to the lateral border of the orbit should be the same on both sides.

63. For the PA axial projection, Haas method, of the skull, where should the central ray enter the patient's head?
    a. Nasion
    b. Acanthion
    c. $1\frac{1}{2}$ inches (3.8 cm) above the external occipital protuberance
    d. $1\frac{1}{2}$ inches (3.8 cm) below the external occipital protuberance

64. How many degrees and in which direction should the central ray be directed for the PA axial projection, Haas method, of the skull?
    a. 15 degrees caudad
    b. 15 degrees cephalad
    c. 25 degrees caudad
    d. 25 degrees cephalad

65. For the parietoorbital oblique projection, Rhese method, of the skull, which positioning line should be perpendicular to the image receptor?
    a. Orbitomeatal
    b. Glabellomeatal
    c. Acanthiomeatal
    d. Infraorbitomeatal

66. For the orbitoparietal oblique projection, Rhese method, of the skull, which positioning line should be perpendicular to the image receptor?
    a. Orbitomeatal
    b. Glabellomeatal
    c. Acanthiomeatal
    d. Infraorbitomeatal

67. With reference to the orbit, where should the optic foramen be imaged on the radiograph to indicate correct positioning of the patient for the parietoorbital oblique projection, Rhese method, of the skull?
    a. Within the lower inner quadrant
    b. Within the lower outer quadrant
    c. Within the upper inner quadrant
    d. Within the upper outer quadrant

68. For the parietoorbital oblique projection, Rhese method, of the skull, how many degrees of angle should be formed between the midsagittal plane and the image receptor?
    a. 25 degrees
    b. 37 degrees
    c. 53 degrees
    d. 55 degrees

69. With reference to the IR, how should the interpupillary line and the midsagittal plane be positioned for the lateral projection to demonstrate the sella turcica?
    a. Interpupillary line: parallel; midsagittal plane: parallel
    b. Interpupillary line: parallel; midsagittal plane: perpendicular
    c. Interpupillary line: perpendicular; midsagittal plane: parallel
    d. Interpupillary line: perpendicular; midsagittal plane: perpendicular

70. For the lateral projection to demonstrate the sella turcica, where should the central ray be directed?
    a. $\frac{3}{4}$ inch (1.9 cm) anterior and $\frac{3}{4}$ inch (1.9 cm) inferior to the external acoustic meatus
    b. $\frac{3}{4}$ inch (1.9 cm) anterior and $\frac{3}{4}$ inch (1.9 cm) superior to the external acoustic meatus
    c. $\frac{3}{4}$ inch (1.9 cm) posterior and $\frac{3}{4}$ inch (1.9 cm) inferior to the external acoustic meatus
    d. $\frac{3}{4}$ inch (1.9 cm) posterior and $\frac{3}{4}$ inch (1.9 cm) superior to the external acoustic meatus

CHAPTER 21

Facial Bones

Radiography of the Facial Bones

Note to students: For a review of facial bone anatomy, see Chapter 20.

Exercise 1: Positioning for Facial Bones and Nasal Bones

Instructions: A standard radiographic series to demonstrate facial bones includes various projections that examine facial structures from different perspectives. Some projections commonly used are the lateral, the parietoacanthial (Waters method), and the acanthioparietal (reverse Waters method). Additionally, a lateral projection of the nasal bones is sometimes added to a facial bones series because nasal bones are sometimes affected when other facial bones are damaged by trauma. This exercise pertains to the projections of the facial bones and nasal bones. Identify structures, fill in missing words, select from a list, or provide a short answer for each item.

Items 1 through 9 pertain to *lateral projections of the facial bones.* Examine Fig. 21-1 as you answer the following items.

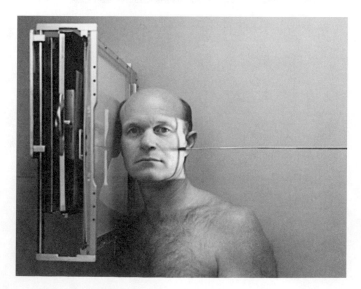

Figure 21-1 Lateral facial bones.

1. The image receptor (IR) should be placed in the IR holder

   _____ (crosswise or lengthwise).

2. The plane of the head that should be parallel with the plane

   of the IR is the _____ (midsagittal or midcoronal) plane.

3. Which positioning line of the head should be perpendicular to the IR?

   a. Orbitomeatal
   b. Interpupillary
   c. Acanthiomeatal
   d. Infraorbitomeatal

4. Which positioning line of the head should be parallel with the transverse axis of the IR?

   a. Orbitomeatal
   b. Interpupillary
   c. Acanthiomeatal
   d. Infraorbitomeatal

5. Which facial bone should be centered to the IR?

   a. Nasal
   b. Maxilla
   c. Mandible
   d. Zygomatic

6. How should the central ray be directed to the patient—perpendicularly, angled cephalically, or angled caudally?

   _____

7. Where on the patient's face should the central ray be directed?

8. From the following list, circle the four evaluation criteria that indicate the patient was properly positioned for a lateral projection of the facial bones.

   a. The sella turcica should not be rotated.
   b. The orbital roofs should be superimposed.
   c. The sella turcica should be seen within the foramen magnum.
   d. The mandibular rami should be almost perfectly superimposed.
   e. The petrous bones should lie in the lower one third of the orbit.
   f. The mental protuberance should be superimposed over anterior frontal bone.
   g. All facial bones should be completely included with the zygomatic bone in the center.
   h. The distance from the lateral border of the skull to the lateral border of the orbit should be equal on both sides.

9. Identify each lettered structure shown in Fig. 21-2.

   A. _____

   B. _____

   C. _____

   D. _____

   E. _____

   F. _____

   G. _____

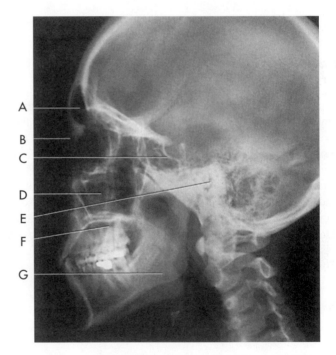

Figure 21-2 Lateral facial bones.

Items 10 through 15 pertain to the *parietoacanthial projection, Waters method.* Examine Fig. 21-3 as you answer the following items.

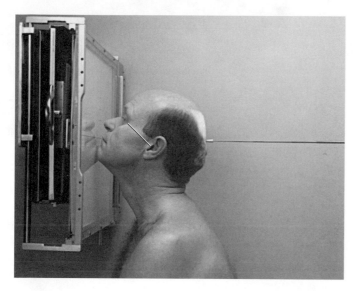

Figure 21-3 Parietoacanthial facial bones, Waters method.

10. Indicate how the orbitomeatal line (OML) and the midsagittal plane should be positioned with reference to the IR.

    a. Orbitomeatal line: _____

    b. Midsagittal plane: _____

11. To which landmark of the head should the IR be centered?
    a. Nasion
    b. Acanthion
    c. Mental point
    d. Outer canthus

12. How should the central ray be directed relative to the IR?
    a. Perpendicularly
    b. 37 degrees caudally
    c. 37 degrees cephalically

13. Describe where the petrous ridges most likely will appear in the image if the orbitomeatal line creates the following angles with the IR:

    a. 25 degrees:

    b. 37 degrees:

    c. 55 degrees:

14. From the following list, circle the two evaluation criteria that indicate the patient was properly positioned for a parietoacanthial projection.
    a. The orbital roofs should be superimposed.
    b. The petrous ridges should nearly fill the orbits.
    c. The entire cranium should be demonstrated without rotation or tilt.
    d. The petrous ridges should be projected immediately below the maxillary sinuses.
    e. The distance between the lateral border of the skull and orbit should be equal on both sides.

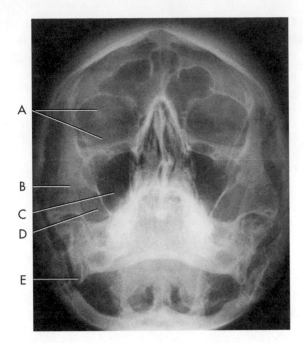

Figure 21-4 Parietoacanthial facial bones, Waters method.

15. Identify each lettered structure shown in Fig. 21-4.

A. _____

B. _____

C. _____

D. _____

E. _____

Items 16 through 24 pertain to the *acanthioparietal projection, reverse Waters method.* Examine Fig. 21-5 as you answer the following items.

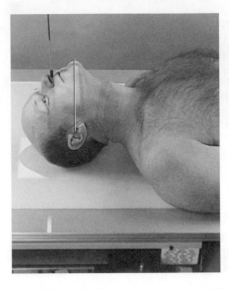

Figure 21-5 Acanthioparietal facial bones, reverse Waters method.

16. The acanthioparietal projection can be used to demonstrate facial bones when the patient is lying in the

_____ (prone or supine) position.

17. The image of the acanthioparietal projection is similar to

the image of the _____ projection

(_____ method).

18. Which plane and positioning line of the head should be perpendicular to the IR?
    a. Midsagittal plane and orbitomeatal line
    b. Midsagittal plane and mentomeatal line
    c. Midcoronal plane and orbitomeatal line
    d. Midcoronal plane and mentomeatal line

19. Where should the midpoint of the IR be centered to the patient?
    a. Nasion
    b. Glabella
    c. Acanthion
    d 1 inch (2.5 cm) inferior to the acanthion

20. Which breathing instructions should be given to the patient?

    a. Stop breathing.
    b. Breathe slowly.
    c. Breathe rapidly.

21. How should the central ray be directed?

    a. Perpendicularly
    b. 15 degrees caudally
    c. 15 degrees cephalically
    d. 30 degrees cephalically

22. To which positioning landmark should the central ray be directed?

    a. Nasion
    b. Glabella
    c. Acanthion
    d. Mental point

23. From the following list, circle the two evaluation criteria that indicate the patient was properly positioned for an acanthioparietal projection, reverse Waters method.

    a. The orbital roofs should be superimposed.
    b. The petrous ridges should nearly fill the orbits.
    c. The petrous ridges should be projected in the maxillary sinuses.
    d. The petrous ridges should be projected immediately below the maxillary sinuses.
    e. The distance between the lateral border of the skull and orbit should be equal on both sides.

24. Identify each lettered structure shown in Fig. 21-6.

    A. _____

    B. _____

    C. _____

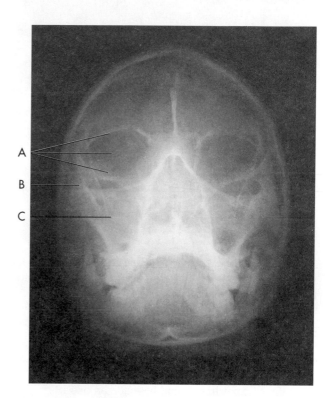

Figure 21-6 Acanthioparietal facial bones, reverse Waters method.

Items 25 through 30 pertain to the *lateral projection of the nasal bones*. Examine Fig. 21-7 as you answer the following items.

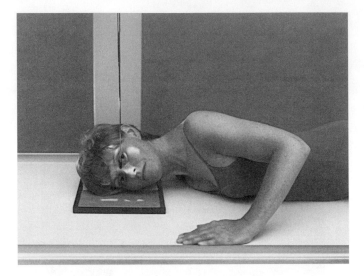

Figure 21-7 Lateral nasal bones.

25. Indicate how the interpupillary line and midsagittal plane should be positioned with reference to the IR—perpendicular or parallel.

   a. Interpupillary line: _____

   b. Midsagittal plane: _____

26. How many exposures should be made on one IR?

   _____

27. To which facial landmark—the nasion or acanthion—should the unmasked portion of the IR be centered?

   _____

28. Describe how and where the central ray should be directed.

29. From the following list, circle the two evaluation criteria that indicate the patient was properly positioned for a lateral projection.

   a All facial bones should be demonstrated.
   b. The zygomatic processes should be seen superimposed.
   c. The anterior nasal spine and frontonasal suture should be visualized.
   d. The nasal bone and soft tissue should be demonstrated without rotation.

30. Identify each lettered structure shown in Fig. 21-8.

   A. _____ (suture)

   B. _____

   C. _____

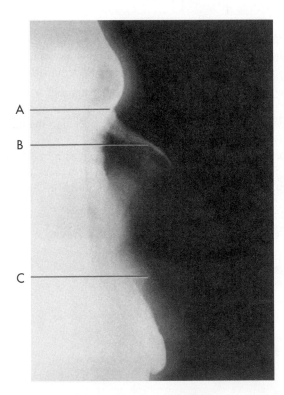

Figure 21-8 Lateral nasal bones.

Exercise 2: Positioning for Zygomatic Arches

Instructions: Zygomatic arches are commonly demonstrated with three projections: a submentovertical (SMV) projection, a tangential projection, and an anteroposterior (AP) axial projection. This exercise pertains to those projections. Identify structures, fill in missing words, provide a short answer, select from a list, or choose true or false (explaining any statement you believe to be false) for each item.

Items 1 through 9 pertain to the *SMV projection for bilateral zygomatic arches*. Examine Fig. 21-9 as you answer the following items.

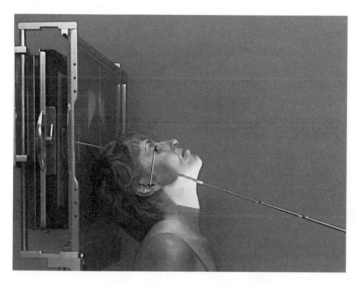

Figure 21-9 SMV zygomatic arches.

1. True or False. The SMV projection should demonstrate both zygomatic arches with one exposure.

2. True or False. Zygomatic arches should be demonstrated superimposed with the anterior frontal bone.

3. True or False. The entire cranial base should be demonstrated.

4. True or False. The midsagittal plane should be parallel with the IR.

5. Which positioning line of the head should be parallel with the IR?
   a. Orbitomeatal
   b. Acanthiomeatal
   c. Infraorbitomeatal

6. Which part of the patient should be in contact with the grid device?
   a. Forehead
   b. Mandible
   c. Vertex of the skull

7. Which statement best describes how the central ray should be directed?
   a. Angled cephalically and centered to the glabella
   b. Angled caudally and centered to the zygomatic arch of interest
   c. Perpendicular to the infraorbitomeatal line and centered on the midsagittal plane of the throat

8. For the SMV projection, what causes the zygomatic arches to be projected beyond the parietal eminences?
   a. The divergent x-ray beam
   b. The head tilted 15 degrees
   c. The head rotated 15 degrees

9. From the following list, circle the three evaluation criteria that indicate the patient was properly positioned for the SMV projection.
   a. No rotation of the head should occur.
   b. The zygomatic arches should be free from overlying structures.
   c. The entire cranium should be demonstrated without rotation or tilt.
   d. The zygomatic arches should be symmetric and without foreshortening.
   e. The structures of the cranial base should be clearly visible as indicated by adequate penetration.
   f. The distance from the lateral border of the skull to the lateral border of the orbit should be equal on both sides.

Items 10 through 14 pertain to the *tangential projection.* Examine Fig. 21-10 as you answer the following items.

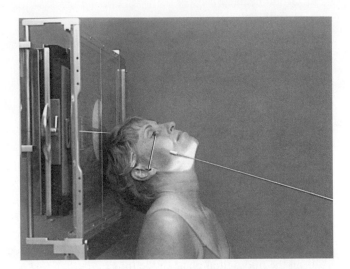

Figure 21-10 Tangential zygomatic arch.

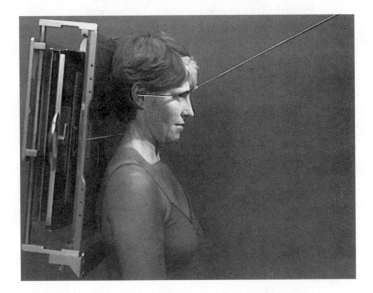

Figure 21-11 AP axial zygomatic arches, modified Towne method.

10. True or False. The patient should hyperextend the neck and rest the head on the vertex.

11. True or False. The midsagittal plane should be perpendicular to the IR.

12. What positioning line of the head should be as parallel as possible with the IR?

13. Describe how the central ray should be directed.

14. From the following list, circle the evaluation criterion that indicates the patient was properly positioned for a tangential projection.
    a. No rotation of the head should occur.
    b. The zygomatic arch should be free from overlying structures.
    c. The entire cranium should be demonstrated without rotation or tilt.

Items 15 through 20 pertain to the *AP axial projection, modified Towne method.* Examine Fig. 21-11 as you answer the following items.

15. Indicate how the orbitomeatal line and midsagittal plane should be positioned with reference to the IR—perpendicular or parallel.

    a. Orbitomeatal line: _____

    b. Midsagittal plane: _____

16. How many degrees and in which direction should the central ray be directed when each of the following positioning lines is placed perpendicular to the plane of the IR?

    a. Orbitomeatal line: _____

    b. Infraorbitomeatal line: _____

17. The central ray should enter 1 inch (2.5 cm) above the

    landmark _____.

18. True or False. Both zygomatic arches should be demonstrated on the radiograph with a single exposure.

19. True or False. The entire vertex should be included on the radiograph.

20. Identify each lettered structure shown in Fig. 21-12.

A. _____

B. _____

C. _____

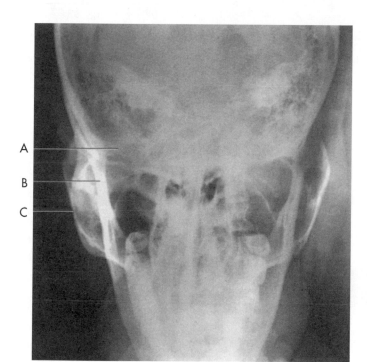

Figure 21-12 AP axial zygomatic arches, modified Towne method.

Exercise 3: Positioning for the Mandible

Instructions: Usually three or four projections are needed to demonstrate the mandible. Posteroanterior (PA), PA axial, and axiolateral oblique projections are often included in the typical mandible examination. This exercise pertains to those projections. Identify structures, provide a short answer, select from a list, or choose true or false (explaining any statement you believe to be false) for each item.

Items 1 through 10 pertain to the *PA projection demonstrating the mandibular rami.* Examine Fig. 21-13 as you answer the following items.

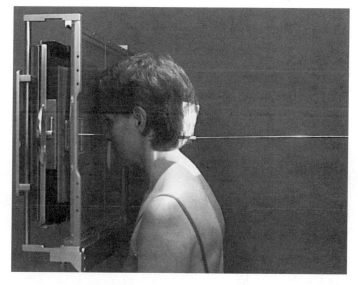

Figure 21-13 PA mandibular rami.

1. To demonstrate the mandibular rami with the PA projection, which two facial structures should be touching the vertical grid device?

   a. Nose and chin
   b. Forehead and nose
   c. Forehead and cheek

2. Which positioning line should be perpendicular to the plane of the IR?

   a. Orbitomeatal
   b. Glabellomeatal
   c. Acanthiomeatal
   d. Infraorbitomeatal

3. How should the midsagittal plane be positioned with reference to the IR—parallel or perpendicular?

4. What breathing instructions should be given to the patient?

5. Through which positioning landmark of the face should the central ray exit?

   a. Nasion
   b. Acanthion
   c. Mental point

6. How does the vertebral column affect the image?

   a. It superimposes mandibular rami.
   b. It superimposes the central part of the mandibular body.
   c. It increases the object-to-IR distance (OID) of the mandible.

7. True or False. The central ray should be directed perpendicularly to the midpoint of the IR.

8. True or False. The PA projection demonstrates the mandibular body without bony superimpositioning.

9. From the following list, circle the two evaluation criteria that indicate the patient was properly positioned for the PA projection of the mandibular rami.

   a. The entire mandible should be included.
   b. The mandibular rami should be superimposed.
   c. The mandibular body and rami should be symmetric on both sides.
   d. The temporomandibular articulation should be seen lying anterior to the external acoustic meatus (EAM).

10. Identify each lettered structure and fracture shown in Fig. 21-14.

    A. _____

    B. _____

    C. _____

    D. _____

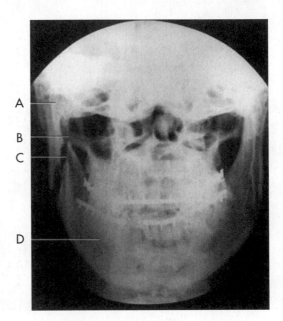

Figure 21-14 PA mandibular rami.

Items 11 through 17 pertain to the *PA axial projection of the mandibular rami.* Examine Fig. 21-15 as you answer the following items.

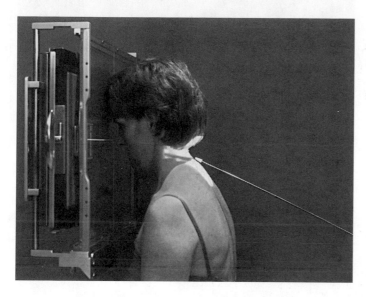

Figure 21-15 PA axial mandibular rami.

11. Which two facial structures should be touching the vertical grid device?

    a. Nose and chin
    b. Forehead and nose
    c. Forehead and cheek

12. Which body plane and positioning line should be perpendicular to the plane of the IR?

    a. Midcoronal plane and orbitomeatal line
    b. Midcoronal plane and acanthiomeatal line
    c. Midsagittal plane and orbitomeatal line
    d. Midsagittal plane and acanthiomeatal line

13. Which breathing instructions should be given to the patient?

    a. Stop breathing.
    b. Breathe slowly.
    c. Breathe rapidly.

14. Which positioning landmark should be centered to the IR?

    a. Nasion
    b. Glabella
    c. Acanthion
    d. Mental point

15. How many degrees and in which direction should the central ray be directed?

    a. 10 to 15 degrees caudad
    b. 10 to 15 degrees cephalad
    c. 20 to 25 degrees caudad
    d. 20 to 25 degrees cephalad

16. What prevents the central part of the mandibular body from being clearly demonstrated?

    a. Superimposition with the spine
    b. Caudal angulation of the central ray
    c. Increased object-to-image receptor distance

17. From the following list, circle the three evaluation criteria that indicate the patient was properly positioned for a PA axial projection.

    a. The entire mandible should be demonstrated.
    b. The mandibular rami should be superimposed.
    c. The condylar processes should be clearly demonstrated.
    d. The mandibular body and rami should be symmetric on both sides.
    e. The temporomandibular articulation should be seen lying anterior to the EAM.

Items 18 through 31 pertain to axiolateral oblique projections of the mandible (with the patient either prone or upright). Figs. 21-16, 21-17, and 21-18 represent three upright axiolateral oblique projections that demonstrate parts of the mandible. Match each of the following positioning statements to one or more of these figures by writing the appropriate figure number in the space provided. Some statements may have more than one figure (projection) associated with them. Some statements do not relate to any of the three projections; answer "NA" for "not applicable" for these items.

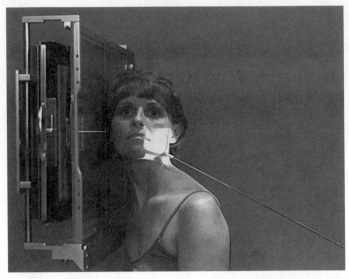

Figure 21-18 Upright axiolateral oblique projection.

_____ 18. Keep the head in a true lateral position.

_____ 19. Used for demonstrating the mandibular body.

_____ 20. Used for demonstrating the mandibular ramus.

_____ 21. Used for demonstrating the mental protuberance.

_____ 22. Rotate the head 30 degrees toward the IR.

_____ 23. Rotate the head 45 degrees toward the IR.

_____ 24. The central ray should exit the mental protuberance.

_____ 25. The central ray should be directed 15 degrees cephalad.

_____ 26. The central ray should be directed 25 degrees cephalad.

_____ 27. The central ray should be directed perpendicular to the IR.

_____ 28. The orbitomeatal line should be perpendicular to the plane of the IR.

_____ 29. The interpupillary line should be perpendicular to the plane of the IR.

_____ 30. The broad surface of the ramus should be parallel with the plane of the IR.

_____ 31. The broad surface of the mandibular body should be parallel with the plane of the IR.

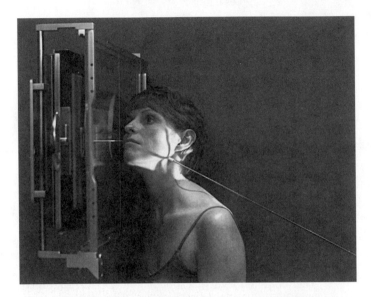

Figure 21-16 Upright axiolateral oblique projection.

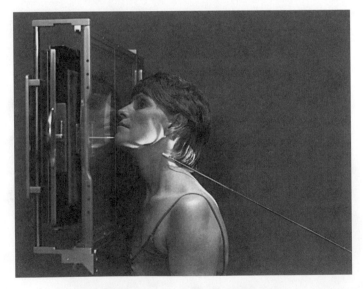

Figure 21-17 Upright axiolateral oblique projection.

32. True or False. The mouth should be closed with the teeth held together.

33. True or False. The neck should be flexed to pull the chin downward.

34. True or False. The area of interest should be parallel with the IR.

35. Identify each lettered structure shown in Fig. 21-19.

A. _____

B. _____

C. _____

D. _____

E. _____

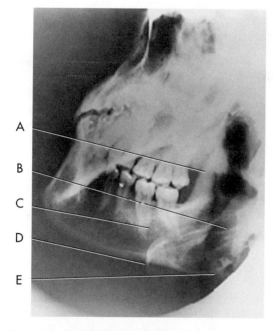

Figure 21-19 Axiolateral oblique mandibular body.

Exercise 4: Positioning for the Temporomandibular Joints (TMJs)

Instructions: Two projections often performed to demonstrate TMJs are the AP axial projection and the axiolateral oblique projection. This exercise pertains to those projections. Identify structures, provide a short answer, select from a list, or choose true or false (explaining any statement you believe to be false) for each question.

Items 1 through 10 pertain to the *AP axial projection.* Examine Fig. 21-20 as you answer the following items.

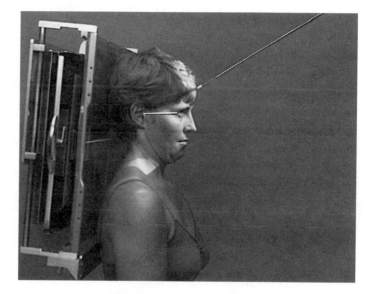

Figure 21-20 AP axial TMJs.

1. True or False. For the AP axial projection in the closed-mouth position, the upper posterior teeth should be in contact with the lower posterior teeth.

2. True or False. The long axis of the mandibular body should be parallel with the transverse axis of the IR.

3. Why should the incisors not contact when the patient is positioned for the closed-mouth AP axial projection?

4. Identify a typical situation in which the patient should not be asked to open his or her mouth wide for an AP axial projection. Explain why.

5. Which plane and positioning line of the head should be perpendicular to the IR?

   a. Midcoronal plane and orbitomeatal line
   b. Midcoronal plane and infraorbitomeatal line
   c. Midsagittal plane and orbitomeatal line
   d. Midsagittal plane and infraorbital meatal line

6. How many degrees and in which direction should the central ray be directed?

   a. 25 degrees caudad
   b. 25 degrees cephalad
   c. 35 degrees caudad
   d. 35 degrees cephalad

7. Where should the central ray enter the patient?

   a. Glabella
   b. Acanthion
   c. 3 inches (7.6 cm) above the nasion
   d. 3 inches (7.6 cm) below the nasion

8. To which landmark should the IR be centered?

   a. Nasion
   b. Glabella
   c. Central ray
   d. Mental protuberance

9. From the following list, circle the two evaluation criteria that indicate the patient was properly positioned for an AP axial projection with the mouth closed.

   a. The head should not be rotated.
   b. The condyle should be seen anterior to the EAM.
   c. Only minimal superimposition by the petrosa on the condyle should be seen.
   d. The condyle and temporomandibular articulation should be seen below the pars petrosa.

10. From the following list, circle the two evaluation criteria that indicate the patient was properly positioned for an AP axial projection with the mouth open.

    a. The head should not be rotated.
    b. The condyle should be seen anterior to the EAM.
    c. Only minimal superimposition by the petrosa on the condyle should be seen.
    d. The condyle and temporomandibular articulation should be demonstrated below the petrosa.

Items 11 through 20 pertain to *axiolateral oblique projections.* Examine Fig. 21-21 as you answer the following items.

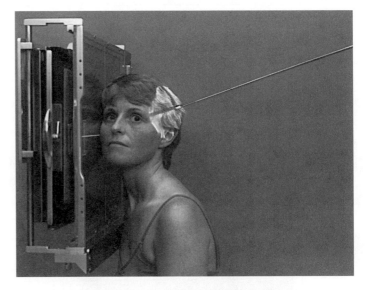

Figure 21-21 Axiolateral oblique TMJ.

11. Where on the patient should the IR be centered?

    a. 2 inches (5 cm) inferior to the TMJs
    b. 2 inches (5 cm) superior to the TMJs
    c. ¹/₂ inch (1.2 cm) anterior to the EAM
    d. ¹/₂ inch (1.2 cm) posterior to the EAM

12. How should the midsagittal plane be positioned with reference to the IR?

    a. Parallel
    b. Perpendicular
    c. Form an angle of 15 degrees
    d. Form an angle of 37 degrees

13. Which positioning line of the head should be parallel with the transverse axis of the IR?

    a. Orbitomeatal
    b. Interpupillary
    c. Acanthiomeatal
    d. Infraorbitomeatal

14. How many degrees and in what direction should the central ray be directed?

_____

15. Through what structure should the central ray exit the patient?

_____

16. In relation to surrounding structures, where in the image should the mandibular condyle be seen for axiolateral oblique projections with the patient holding the mouth closed?

_____

17. True or False. The central ray should enter the patient at the TMJ farther from the IR.

18. True or False. Both open- and closed-mouth positions should be performed with the axiolateral oblique projection unless contraindicated.

19. True or False. The entire side of the mandible from the condyle to the symphysis should be demonstrated.

20. Identify each lettered structure shown in Fig. 21-22.

A. _____

B. _____

C. _____

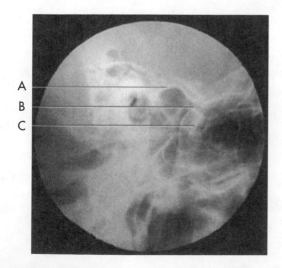

Figure 21-22 Axiolateral oblique TMJ with the patient's mouth open.

Exercise 5: Evaluating Radiographs of Facial Bones

Instructions: This exercise consists of facial bone radiographs to give you some practice evaluating facial bone positioning. These images are not from _Merrill's Atlas of Radiographic Positions and Radiologic Procedures._ Most images show at least one positioning error. Examine each image and answer the questions that follow by providing a short answer.

1. Fig. 21-23 shows a lateral projection radiograph of the facial bones with incorrect positioning of a phantom skull. Examine the image and state why it does not meet the evaluation criteria for this type of projection.

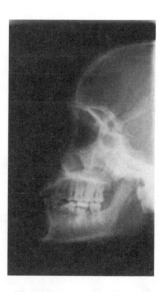

Figure 21-23 Lateral facial bones showing incorrect positioning of a phantom skull.

2. Figs. 21-24 through 21-26 show parietoacanthial projection radiographs of the facial bones of a phantom skull. Only one image demonstrates acceptable positioning. Examine the images and answer the questions that follow.

a. Which image demonstrates acceptable positioning?

_____

b. In which image does the phantom skull appear to be incorrectly positioned because the angle between the OML and the IR is greater than the required amount? (This error results when the patient is unable to extend the neck far enough.)

_____

c. In which image does the phantom skull appear to be incorrectly positioned because the angle between the OML and the IR is less than the required amount? (This error results when the patient extends the neck too much.)

_____

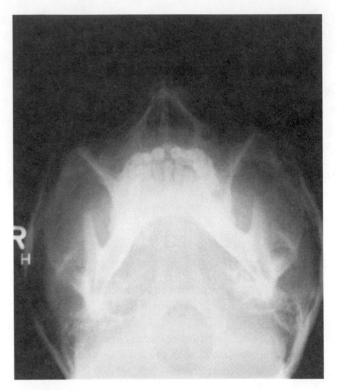

Figure 21-25 Radiograph of a phantom skull positioned for the parietoacanthial projection.

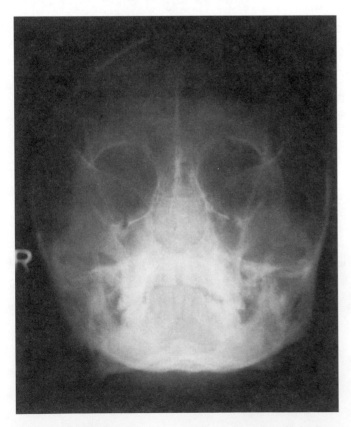

Figure 21-24 Radiograph of a phantom skull positioned for the parietoacanthial projection.

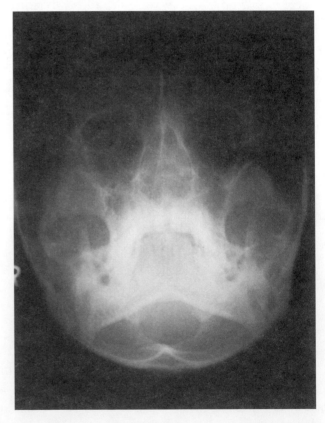

Figure 21-26 Radiograph of a phantom skull positioned for the parietoacanthial projection.

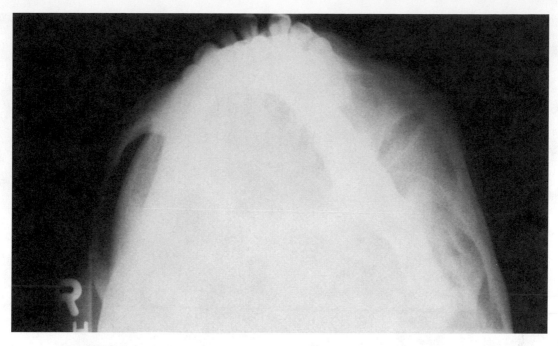

Figure 21-27 SMV projection of a phantom skull for zygomatic arches.

3. Fig. 21-27 shows a submentovertical projection radiograph of the zygomatic arches with incorrect positioning of a phantom skull. Examine the image and answer the questions that follow.

a. What image characteristics prevent the image from meeting all evaluation criteria for this projection?

b. What positioning error most likely resulted in this unacceptable image?

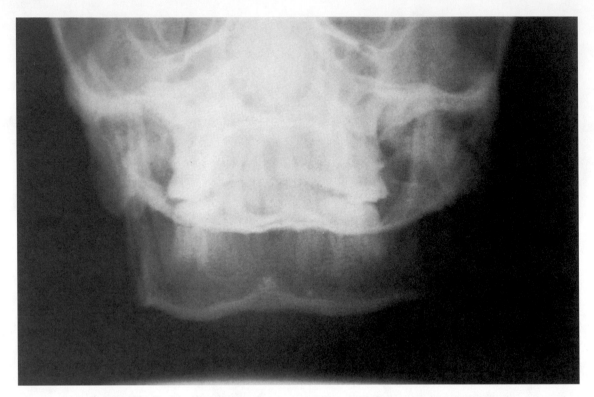

Figure 21-28 PA mandibular rami showing incorrect positioning of a phantom skull.

4. Fig. 21-28 shows a PA projection radiograph demonstrating the mandibular rami with incorrect positioning of a phantom skull. Examine the image and answer the questions that follow.

   a. What image characteristic prevents this radiograph from being of acceptable quality?

   b. To comply with the evaluation criteria for this projection, how should the position of the phantom skull be adjusted for a subsequent radiograph?

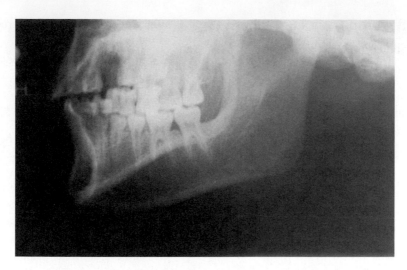

Figure 21-29 Axiolateral oblique mandibular body showing incorrect positioning of a phantom skull.

5. Fig. 21-29 shows an axiolateral oblique projection radiograph of the mandibular body with incorrect positioning of a phantom skull. Examine the image and answer the questions that follow.

a. What image characteristic prevents the image from meeting all evaluation criteria for this type of projection?

b. How should the position of the phantom skull be adjusted for a subsequent radiograph?

Note to Students: Additional exercises referenced from Chapters 20 through 23 are found in the Appendix (Supplemental Exercises for Skull Positioning), which is located in this workbook. Students should complete the review exercises for those chapters before completing the appendix exercises.

Self-Test: Radiography of the Facial Bones

Instructions: Answer the following questions by selecting the best choice.

1. With reference to the patient, where should the central ray be directed for the lateral projection of the facial bones?

   a. Zygoma
   b. Nasal bones
   c. Outer canthus
   d. $^3/_4$ inch (1.9 cm) anterior and $^3/_4$ inch (1.9 cm) superior to the EAM

2. With reference to the IR, how should the central ray be directed for the parietoacanthial projection, Waters method?

   a. Perpendicular
   b. 15 degrees caudad
   c. 23 degrees caudad
   d. 37 degrees caudad

3. Where should the petrous ridges be seen in the image of the parietoacanthial projection of the facial bones?

   a. Superior to the orbits
   b. Lower one third of the orbits
   c. Through the maxillary sinuses
   d. Below the maxillary sinuses

4. Which positioning line and angle indicate correct positioning of the head for the parietoacanthial projection, Waters method?

   a. Orbitomeatal line; 37 degrees to the IR
   b. Orbitomeatal line; perpendicular to the IR
   c. Infraorbitomeatal line; 37 degrees to the IR
   d. Infraorbitomeatal line; perpendicular to the IR

5. Which evaluation criterion pertains to the parietoacanthial projection, Waters method?

   a. The orbital roofs should be superimposed.
   b. The petrous ridges should be projected within the orbits.
   c. The zygomatic arches should be free from overlying structures.
   d. The petrous ridges should be projected immediately below the maxillary sinuses.

6. Which evaluation criterion pertains to the parietoacanthial projection, Waters method?

   a. The orbital roofs should be superimposed.
   b. The zygomatic arches should be superimposed.
   c. The petrous pyramids should be projected within the orbits.
   d. The distance between the lateral border of the skull and orbit should be the same on both sides.

7. Which evaluation criterion pertains to the lateral projection of the facial bones?

   a. The orbital roofs should be superimposed.
   b. The petrous ridges should be projected within the orbits.
   c. The zygomatic arches should be free from overlying structures.
   d. The petrous ridges should be projected immediately below the maxillary sinuses.

8. Which evaluation criterion pertains to the SMV projection for bilateral zygomatic arches?

   a. The orbital roofs should be superimposed.
   b. The zygomatic arches should be superimposed.
   c. The petrous ridges should be projected within the orbits.
   d. The zygomatic arches should be free from overlying structures.

9. An AP axial projection (modified Towne method) of the bilateral zygomatic arches produces an image similar to the AP axial projection (Towne method) of the skull. How many degrees and in what direction should the central ray be directed for this projection to demonstrate zygomatic arches when the OML is perpendicular to the IR?

   a. 30 degrees caudad
   b. 37 degrees caudad
   c. 30 degrees cephalad
   d. 37 degrees cephalad

10. An AP axial projection (modified Towne method) of the bilateral zygomatic arches is performed similarly to the AP axial projection (Towne method) of the skull, except that the projection for the zygomatic arches requires that which of the following be done?

    a. The central ray should be directed cephalically.
    b. The central ray should be directed to the glabella.
    c. The orbitomeatal line forms an angle of 37 degrees with the IR.
    d. The midsagittal plane forms an angle of 45 degrees with the IR.

11. With reference to the IR, how should the midsagittal plane be adjusted for the tangential projection demonstrating an individual zygomatic arch?

    a. Parallel with the IR
    b. 15 degrees from perpendicular
    c. 37 degrees to the IR
    d. 53 degrees to the IR

12. To demonstrate the mandibular body with the axiolateral oblique projection, how should the patient's head be positioned?

    a. Keep the head in a true lateral position.
    b. From true lateral, rotate the head 15 degrees toward the IR.
    c. From true lateral, rotate the head 30 degrees toward the IR.
    d. From true lateral, rotate the head 45 degrees toward the IR.

13. How many degrees and in which direction should the central ray be directed for the axiolateral oblique projection of the mandible?

    a. 15 degrees caudad
    b. 15 degrees cephalad
    c. 25 degrees caudad
    d. 25 degrees cephalad

14. Which projection is performed with the patient's head positioned true lateral and the central ray directed 25 degrees cephalad?

    a. Axiolateral oblique projections of the TMJs
    b. Axiolateral oblique projections of the mandible
    c. Parietoacanthial projections of the facial bones
    d. Tangential projections of the bilateral zygomatic arches

15. Which evaluation criterion pertains to the axiolateral oblique projection of the mandible?

    a. The mandibular rami should be superimposed.
    b. The opposite side of the mandible should not overlap the ramus.
    c. The mandibular condyles should be anterior to the petrous ridges.
    d. The mental protuberance should superimpose anterior frontal bone.

16. Which structure is of primary interest when the patient's head is rotated 15 degrees toward the IR from a true lateral position and the central ray is directed 15 degrees caudad, entering about $1\frac{1}{2}$ inches (3.8 cm) superior to the upside EAM?

    a. Orbit
    b. Mandible
    c. Zygomatic arch
    d. Temporomandibular joint

17. Which of the following structures can be well demonstrated with an axiolateral oblique projection?

    a. Facial bones
    b. Zygomatic arches
    c. Maxillary sinuses
    d. Temporomandibular joints

18. How many degrees and in which direction should the central ray be directed for the axiolateral oblique projection for TMJs?

    a. 15 degrees caudad
    b. 15 degrees cephalad
    c. 25 degrees caudad
    d. 25 degrees cephalad

19. For the AP axial projection of the TMJs, where should the central ray be directed?

    a. Nasion
    b. Glabella
    c. Acanthion
    d. 3 inches (7.6 cm) above the nasion

20. With reference to the patient, where should the IR be centered for the axiolateral oblique projection of the TMJs?

    a. To the glabella
    b. $\frac{1}{2}$ inch (1.2 cm) anterior to the EAM
    c. 1 inch (2.5 cm) posterior to the EAM
    d. 2 inches (5 cm) above the EAM

CHAPTER 23

Temporal Bone

Review

Note to students: For a review of the temporal bone anatomy, see Chapter 20.

Instructions: Although computed tomography (CT) is often used to image internal cranial structures, small medical facilities still use standard radiography to demonstrate the mastoid processes and petrous portions. The axiolateral projections (modified Law method, single-tube angulation) can be used to image mastoid air cells, and both axiolateral oblique projections (Stenvers method, posterior profile, and Arcelin method, anterior profile) can be used to demonstrate petrous portions. This exercise pertains to those types of projections. Identify structures, provide a short answer, select from a list, or choose true or false (explaining any statement you believe to be false) for each item.

Items 1 through 11 pertain to the *axiolateral projection (modified Law method, single-tube angulation).* Examine Fig. 23-1 as you answer the following items.

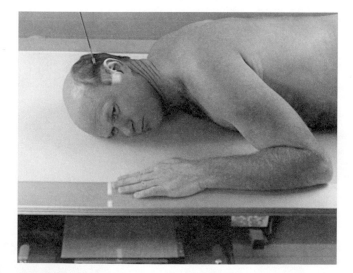

Figure 23-1 Axiolateral petromastoid portion (modified Law method, single-tube angulation).

1. Describe how the patient's head should be positioned.

2. Which procedure should be performed to prevent soft-tissue structures from overlapping the mastoid process of interest?
   a. Tape the auricle of the ear forward.
   b. Angle the central ray 25 degrees caudad.
   c. Angle the central ray 25 degrees cephalad.
   d. Rotate the patient's head until the midsagittal plane forms an angle of 30 degrees with the plane of the image receptor (IR).

3. If the patient is rotated 15 degrees from the right lateral position, which mastoid—right or left—is of interest? Is it the side closer to or farther from the image receptor?
   a. Left side; closer to
   b. Left side; farther from
   c. Right side; closer to
   d. Right side; farther from

4. Where should the IR be centered to the patient?
   a. 2 inches (5 cm) above the external acoustic meatus (EAM)
   b. 2 inches (5 cm) below the EAM
   c. 1 inch (2.5 cm) anterior to the EAM of the side adjacent to the IR
   d. 1 inch (2.5 cm) posterior to the EAM of the side adjacent to the IR

5. How many degrees and in what direction should the central ray be directed?

6. Where should the central ray enter the patient?

7. True or False. The patient's head should be placed and kept in the true lateral position.

8. True or False. The patient's head should be rotated from the true anteroposterior (AP) position until the midsagittal plane forms an angle of 15 degrees from vertical.

9. True or False. The interpupillary line should remain perpendicular to the IR throughout the positioning procedure.

10. From the following list, circle the six evaluation criteria that indicate the patient was properly positioned for an axiolateral projection (modified Law method, single-tube angulation).

    a. Close beam restriction of the mastoid region is needed.
    b. The auricle of the ear should not superimpose the mastoid.
    c. The entire side of the cranium should be clearly demonstrated.
    d. The petrous ridges should superimpose the mastoid of interest.
    e. The mastoid process should be in profile below the margin of the cranium.
    f. The internal and external acoustic meatuses should be superimposed.
    g. The temporomandibular joint should be visualized anterior to the mastoid.
    h. The temporomandibular joint should be visualized posterior to the mastoid.
    i. The opposite mastoid should not superimpose but should lie inferior and slightly anterior to the mastoid of interest.
    j. The mastoid closer to the IR should be included, and the air cells should be demonstrated and centered to the IR.

11. Identify each lettered structure shown in Fig. 23-2.

A. _____   C. _____

B. _____   D. _____

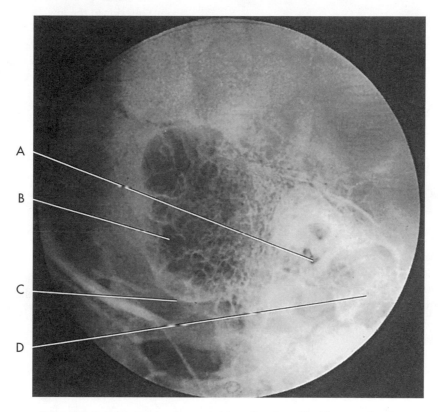

Figure 23-2 Axiolateral petromastoid portion (modified Law method).

Items 12 through 18 pertain to the *axiolateral oblique projection (Stenvers method, posterior profile)*. Examine Fig. 23-3 as you answer the following items.

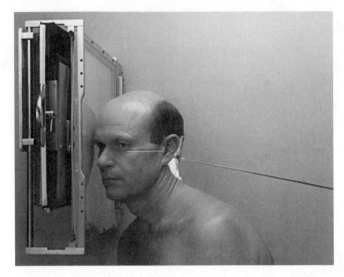

Figure 23-3 Axiolateral oblique petromastoid portion (Stenvers method), posterior profile.

12. What three points of the face should be in contact with the x-ray table or vertical grid device?

13. How many degrees and in what direction should the central ray be directed?

14. Where on the head should the central ray enter the patient?
   a. 2 inches (5 cm) above the EAM
   b. 2 inches (5 cm) below the EAM
   c. 3 to 4 inches (7.6 to 10 cm) anterior and $1/2$ inch (1.2 cm) superior to the upside EAM
   d. 3 to 4 inches (7.6 to 10 cm) posterior and $1/2$ inch (1.2 cm) inferior to the upside EAM

15. The midsagittal plane with the plane of the image receptor should form an angle of how many degrees?
   a. 15 degrees
   b. 37 degrees
   c. 45 degrees
   d. 53 degrees

16. Which positioning line of the head should be parallel with the transverse axis of the image receptor?
   a. Orbitomeatal
   b. Interpupillary
   c. Acanthiomeatal
   d. Infraorbitomeatal

17. Which petrous pyramid is demonstrated in profile when the patient is facing toward the left shoulder, as shown in Fig. 23-3? Is it the petrous pyramid closer to or farther from the image receptor?
   a. Left side; closer to
   b. Left side; farther from
   c. Right side; closer to
   d. Right side; farther from

18. Identify each lettered structure shown in Fig. 23-4.

A. _____   D. _____

B. _____   E. _____

C. _____   F. _____

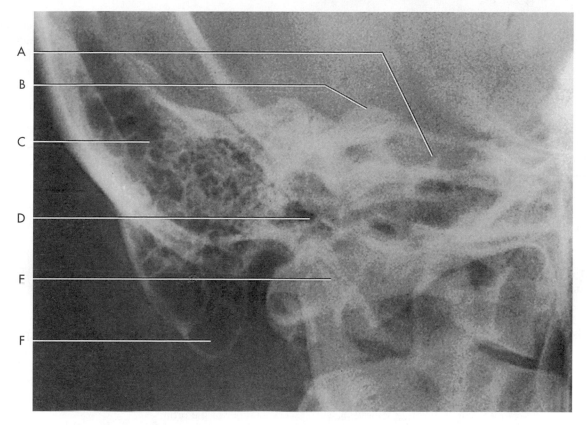

Figure 23-4 Axiolateral oblique petromastoid portion (Stenvers method), posterior profile.

Items 19 through 25 pertain to the *axiolateral oblique projection (Arcelin method, anterior profile)*. Examine Fig. 23-5 as you answer the following items.

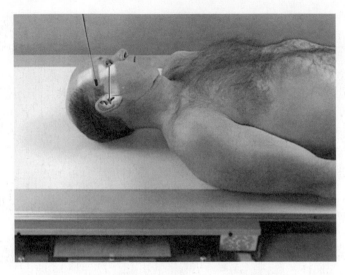

Figure 23-5 Axiolateral oblique petromastoid portion (Arcelin method), anterior profile.

19. True or False. The patient should be placed in the supine position.

20. True or False. The midsagittal plane should be perpendicular to the image receptor.

21. True or False. The infraorbitomeatal line should be perpendicular to the image receptor.

22. How many degrees and in what direction should the central ray be directed?

23. Where should the central ray enter the patient?

24. Which petrous pyramid—right or left—is demonstrated in profile when the patient is facing toward the left shoulder, as shown in Fig. 23-5? Is it the petrous pyramid closer to or farther from the image receptor?

    a. Left side; closer to
    b. Left side; farther from
    c. Right side; closer to
    d. Right side; farther from

25. From the following list, circle the six evaluation criteria that indicate the patient was properly positioned for either a posterior profile projection (Stenvers method) or an anterior profile projection (Arcelin method).

    a. The petrous ridges should completely fill the orbits.
    b. The petromastoid portion should be demonstrated in profile.
    c. The entire side of the cranium should be clearly demonstrated.
    d. The internal and external acoustic meatuses should be superimposed.
    e. The lateral border of the skull to the lateral border of the orbit should be included.
    f. The mastoid should be demonstrated in profile below the margin of the cranium.
    g. The mandibular condyle should be projected over the first cervical vertebra near the petrosa.
    h. The posterior surface of the ramus should parallel or superimpose the lateral surface of the cervical vertebrae.
    i. The opposite mastoid should not superimpose, but should lie inferior and slightly anterior to the mastoid of interest.
    j. The petrous ridge should lie horizontally and at a point approximately two thirds of the way up the lateral border of the orbit.
    k. The mastoid closer to the image receptor should be included, with the air cells demonstrated and centered to the IR.

Note to Students: Additional exercises referenced from Chapters 20 through 23 are found in the Appendix (Supplemental Exercises for Skull Positioning), which is located in this workbook. Students should complete the review exercises for those chapters before completing the appendix exercises.

Self-Test: Radiography of the Temporal Bone

Instructions: Answer the following questions by selecting the best choice.

1. Which projection method produces an axiolateral view of a mastoid?

    a. Waters method
    b. Arcelin method
    c. Stenvers method
    d. Modified Law method

2. Which projection requires that the central ray be directed 15 degrees caudad?

    a. Parietoacanthial (Waters method)
    b. Axiolateral oblique (Arcelin method, anterior profile)
    c. Axiolateral oblique (Stenvers method, posterior profile)
    d. Axiolateral (modified Law method, single-tube angulation)

3. Which projection requires that the patient's head be rotated from true lateral, moving the face closer to the IR, until the midsagittal plane forms an angle of 15 degrees with the IR?

    a. Parietoacanthial (Waters method)
    b. Axiolateral oblique (Arcelin method, anterior profile)
    c. Axiolateral oblique (Stenvers method, posterior profile)
    d. Axiolateral (modified Law method, single-tube angulation)

4. Which projection requires that the central ray enter at a point 2 inches (5 cm) posterior to and 2 inches (5 cm) superior to the uppermost EAM?

    a. Parietoacanthial (Waters method)
    b. Axiolateral oblique (Arcelin method, anterior profile)
    c. Axiolateral oblique (Stenvers method, posterior profile)
    d. Axiolateral (modified Law method, single-tube angulation)

5. For axiolateral projections (modified Law method, single-tube angulation), how many degrees and in which direction should the central ray be directed?

    a. 10 degrees caudad
    b. 10 degrees cephalad
    c. 15 degrees caudad
    d. 15 degrees cephalad

6. Which structure is best demonstrated when the patient's head is rotated from true left lateral, moving the face closer to the IR until the midsagittal plane forms an angle of 15 degrees with the plane of the IR, and the central ray is directed caudally to exit the skull 1 inch (2.5 cm) posterior to the EAM?

    a. Left petrous portion
    b. Right petrous portion
    c. Left mastoid air cells
    d. Right mastoid air cells

7. If the patient is rotated 15 degrees from the left lateral position when performing the axiolateral projection (modified Law method, single-tube angulation), which mastoid is of interest? Is it the side closer to or farther from the IR?

    a. Left side; closer to
    b. Left side; farther from
    c. Right side; closer to
    d. Right side; farther from

8. Which evaluation criterion pertains to the axiolateral projection (modified Law method, single-tube angulation)?

    a. The petrous ridges should lie in the lower one third of both orbits.
    b. The petrous ridges should be demonstrated in profile without distortion.
    c. The mastoid process should be projected below the shadow of the occipital bone.
    d. The mastoid closer to the IR should be included, with the air cells demonstrated and centered to the IR.

9. How many degrees and in which direction should the central ray be directed for axiolateral oblique projections (Stenvers method, posterior profile)?

    a. 10 degrees caudad
    b. 10 degrees cephalad
    c. 12 degrees caudad
    d. 12 degrees cephalad

10. How many degrees and in which direction should the central ray be directed for axiolateral oblique projections (Arcelin method, anterior profile)?

    a. 10 degrees caudad
    b. 10 degrees cephalad
    c. 12 degrees caudad
    d. 12 degrees cephalad

11. Which evaluation criterion pertains to the axiolateral oblique projection (Stenvers method, posterior profile)?

   a. The petrous ridge should lie in the lower one third of the orbit.
   b. The petromastoid portion should be demonstrated in profile without distortion.
   c. The mastoid process should be projected below the shadow of the occipital bone.
   d. The mastoid closer to the IR should be included, with the air cells demonstrated and centered to the IR.

12. Which projection requires that the patient's head be rotated from the PA position until the midsagittal plane forms an angle of 45 degrees with the IR and that the central ray be directed to exit the skull 1 inch (2.5 cm) anterior to the EAM?

   a. Tangential for individual zygomatic arches
   b. Axiolateral oblique (Arcelin method, anterior profile)
   c. Axiolateral oblique (Stenvers method, posterior profile)
   d. Axiolateral (modified Law method, single-tube angulation)

13. Which projection requires that the patient's head be rotated from the AP position until the midsagittal plane forms an angle of 45 degrees with the plane of the IR and that the central ray be directed to enter the side of the face at a point about 1 inch (2.5 cm) anterior and $^3/_4$ inch (1.9 cm) superior to the EAM?

   a. Submentovertical (Schüller method)
   b. Axiolateral oblique (Arcelin method, anterior profile)
   c. Axiolateral oblique (Stenvers method, posterior profile)
   d. Axiolateral (modified Law method, single-tube angulation)

14. Which structure is best demonstrated when the patient's head is rotated from the PA position, moving the occipital bone closer to the right shoulder, until the midsagittal plane forms an angle of 45 degrees with the plane of the IR and the central ray is directed to exit the skull 1 inch (2.5 cm) anterior to the EAM?

   a. Left petrous portion
   b. Right petrous portion
   c. Left mastoid air cells
   d. Right mastoid air cells

15. Which structure is best demonstrated when the patient's head is rotated from the AP position, moving the face toward the right shoulder, until the midsagittal plane forms an angle of 45 degrees with the plane of the IR, and the central ray is directed to enter the side of the face about 1 inch (2.5 cm) anterior and $^3/_4$ inch (1.9 cm) superior to the EAM?

   a. Left petrous portion
   b. Right petrous portion
   c. Left mastoid air cells
   d. Right mastoid air cells

CHAPTER 24

Mammography

SECTION 1

Anatomy and Physiology of the Breast

Exercise 1

Instructions: This exercise pertains to the anatomy of the breast. Identify structures for each illustration.

1. Identify each lettered structure shown in Fig. 24-1.

   A. _____

   B. _____

   C. _____

   D. _____

2. Identify each lettered structure shown in Fig. 24-2.

   A. _____

   B. _____

   C. _____

   D. _____

   E. _____

   F. _____

   G. _____

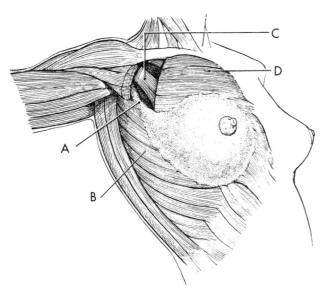

Figure 24-1 Relationship of the breast to the chest wall.

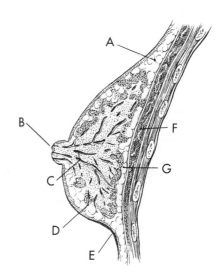

Figure 24-2 Sagittal section through the breast illustrating structural anatomy.

Exercise 2

1. Another term for the female breast is the

   _____ gland.

2. The female breast functions as an accessory gland to the reproductive system by producing and secreting

   _____.

3. The axillary prolongation of the breast is also called the

   axillary _____.

4. The posterior surface of the breast overlying the muscles is

   the _____.

5. The female breast tapers anteriorly from the base, ending

   in the _____.

6. The circular area of pigmented skin that surrounds the nip-

   ple is the _____.

7. The adult female breast contains _____

   to _____ lobes.

8. The glandular elements found in the lobules of the female

   breast are the _____.

9. As a female gets older, the size of her breast lobules be-

   comes _____.

10. The normal process of change in breast tissues that occurs

    as the patient ages is termed _____.

11. Normal involution replaces glandular and parenchymal tis-
    sues with increased amounts of

    _____.

12. The ducts that drain milk from the lobes are the

    _____ ducts.

13. Another term for the suspensory ligaments of the breast is

    _____ ligaments.

14. Approximately 75% of the lymph drainage is toward the

    _____.

15. The internal mammary lymph nodes are situated behind

    the _____.

Exercise 3

Match the pathology terms in Column A with the appropriate definition in Column B. Not all choices from Column B should be selected.

Column A	Column B
____ 1. Cyst	a. Narrowing or contraction of a passage
____ 2. Tumor	b. Formation of fibrous tissue in the breast
____ 3. Fibrosis	c. Proliferation of the epithelium of the breast
____ 4. Carcinoma	d. A benign, neoplastic papillary growth in a duct
____ 5. Calcification	e. Malignant new growth composed of epithelial cells
____ 6. Fibroadenoma	f. Benign tumor of the breast containing fibrous elements
____ 7 Intraductal papilloma	g. New tissue growth in which cell proliferation is uncontrolled
____ 8. Epithelial hyperplasia	h. Closed epithelial sac containing fluid or a semisolid substance
	i. Deposit of calcium salt in tissue; characteristics may suggest either benign or malignant processes

SECTION 2

Radiography of the Breast

Exercise 1

Instructions: Mammography is used to demonstrate diseases of the breast. This exercise pertains to mammographic procedures. Provide a short answer or select from a list for each question.

1. Why should the breast be bared for the examination?

2. Why should the patient remove deodorant and powder from the axilla?

3. Name the two standard projections routinely performed to demonstrate the breast.

4. What condition requires that a nipple marker be placed on the patient?

5. What procedure should a radiographer perform to help produce uniform breast thickness?

6. What procedure should a radiographer perform to identify the location of a palpable mass?

7. Why should the posterior nipple line be measured and compared between two projections?

8. Between what two structures should the posterior nipple line be measured in craniocaudal projections?

9. What is the maximum difference for the length of the posterior nipple line when comparing images of craniocaudal and mediolateral oblique projections?

10. Between examinations, what should a radiographer do to the image receptor (IR) surface and face guard?

Exercise 2

Instructions: Identify each of the following four illustrations of mammography projections by selecting the best choice from the list provided for each illustration.

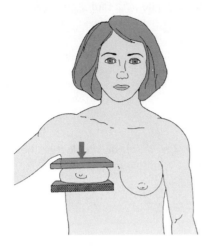

Figure 24-3 Illustration of a mammographic projection.

1. Fig. 24-3
   a. Craniocaudal
   b. Mediolateral
   c. Mediolateral oblique
   d. Exaggerated craniocaudal

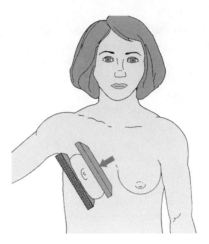

Figure 24-5 Illustration of a mammographic projection.

3. Fig. 24-5
   a. Craniocaudal
   b. Mediolateral
   c. Mediolateral oblique
   d. Exaggerated craniocaudal

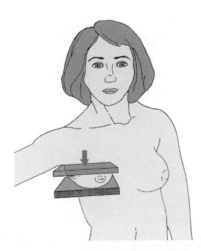

Figure 24-4 Illustration of a mammographic projection.

2. Fig. 24-4
   a. Craniocaudal
   b. Mediolateral
   c. Mediolateral oblique
   d. Exaggerated craniocaudal

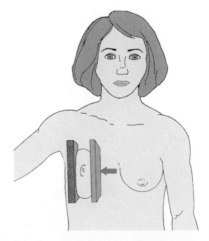

Figure 24-6 Illustration of a mammographic projection.

4. Fig. 24-6
   a. Craniocaudal
   b. Mediolateral
   c. Mediolateral oblique
   d. Exaggerated craniocaudal

Exercise 3

Items 1 through 10 are statements that refer to mammography positioning procedures. Examine each statement in Column A and identify the mammography projection from Column B that most closely relates to the statement. Some statements pertain to more than one projection.

Column A

_____ 1. The breast should be perpendicular to the chest wall.

_____ 2. Slowly apply compression until the breast feels taut.

_____ 3. Elevate the inframammary fold to its maximum height.

_____ 4. Direct the central ray perpendicular to the base of the breast.

_____ 5. Direct the central ray 5 degrees mediolaterally to the base of the breast.

_____ 6. Instruct the patient to stand or be seated facing the IR holder.

_____ 7. Rotate the C-arm to direct the central ray to the medial side of the breast.

_____ 8. Adjust the height of the IR to the level of the inferior surface of the breast.

_____ 9. Adjust the height of the IR so that the superior border is level with the axilla.

_____ 10. Pull the breast tissue superiorly and anteriorly, ensuring that the lateral rib margin is firmly pressed against the IR.

Column B

a. Mediolateral

b. Craniocaudal

c. Mediolateral oblique

d. Exaggerated craniocaudal

Exercise 4

Items 1 through 8 are statements that refer to structures that are demonstrated with various mammography projections. Examine each statement in Column A and identify the mammography projection from Column B that most closely relates to the statement.

Column A

_____ 1. Demonstrates air-fluid and fat-fluid levels in breast structures.

_____ 2. Resolves superimposed structures seen on the MLO projection.

_____ 3. Demonstrates the pectoral muscle approximately 30% of the time.

_____ 4. Demonstrates all breast tissue with emphasis on the lateral aspect and axillary tail.

_____ 5. The central, subareolar, and medial fibroglandular breast tissue should be demonstrated.

_____ 6. Demonstrates lesions on the lateral aspect of the breast in the superior or inferior aspects.

_____ 7. Demonstrates a sagittal orientation of a lateral lesion located in the axillary tail of the breast.

_____ 8. Demonstrates a superoinferior projection of the lateral fibroglandular breast tissue and posterior aspect of the pectoral muscle.

Column B

a. Mediolateral

b. Craniocaudal

c. Mediolateral oblique

d. Exaggerated craniocaudal

Self-Test: Mammography

Instructions: Answer the following questions by selecting the best choice.

1. The lymphatic vessels of the breast drain laterally into which of the following lymph nodes?

   a. Axillary
   b. Thoracic
   c. Abdominal
   d. Internal mammary chain

2. Where is the tail of the breast located?

   a. Adjacent to the nipple
   b. Along the lateral side to the axilla
   c. Along the medial aspect of the breast
   d. In the glandular tissue against the chest wall

3. Which ducts drain milk from the lobes of the breast?

   a. Axillary
   b. Thoracic
   c. Lymphatic
   d. Lactiferous

4. How do breast tissues change after involution?

   a. Glandular tissues become dense and opaque.
   b. Parenchymal tissues become dense and opaque.
   c. Fatty tissues are replaced with glandular tissues.
   d. Glandular tissues are replaced with fatty tissues.

5. Which two projections comprise the standard examination for demonstrating the breasts?

   a. Craniocaudal and lateromedial
   b. Craniocaudal and mediolateral oblique
   c. Caudocranial and lateromedial
   d. Caudocranial and mediolateral oblique

6. Which projection requires that the central ray pass through the breast at an angle of 30 to 60 degrees?

   a. Axillary
   b. Caudocranial
   c. Craniocaudal
   d. Mediolateral oblique

7. Which muscle is often demonstrated with the craniocaudal projection?

   a. Pectoralis major
   b. Serratus anterior
   c. Rectus abdominis
   d. Lateral abdominal oblique

8. What is the primary objective of compressing the breast for mammography?

   a. To reduce exposure time
   b. To decrease geometric distortion
   c. To produce uniform breast thickness
   d. To produce uniform radiographic density

9. Where should the radiopaque marker, used to indicate which side is being examined, be seen on the image of craniocaudal projections?

   a. On the nipple
   b. On the chest wall
   c. Along the lateral side of the breast
   d. Along the medial side of the breast

10. How should a radiographer identify the location of a palpable mass?

    a. Draw a circle around the mass on the resultant mammogram.
    b. Use an ink marker to draw a circle on the skin overlying the mass.
    c. Place a radiopaque marker such as a BB on the breast overlying the mass.
    d. Place a radiopaque arrow marker alongside the breast to point to the mass.

11. What is the maximum difference for the length of the posterior nipple line when comparing images of craniocaudal and mediolateral oblique projections?

    a. 0.5 cm
    b. 1.0 cm
    c. 1.5 cm
    d. 2.0 cm

12. Between which two projections should the posterior nipple lines be measured and compared?

    a. Craniocaudal and mediolateral oblique
    b. Craniocaudal and 90-degree mediolateral
    c. Exaggerated craniocaudal and mediolateral oblique
    d. Exaggerated craniocaudal and 90-degree mediolateral

13. In which body position should the patient be placed for craniocaudal or mediolateral oblique projections?

    a. Prone
    b. Supine
    c. Upright
    d. Lateral recumbent

14. Which projection demonstrates all breast tissue with an emphasis on the lateral aspect and axillary tail?

    a. Mediolateral
    b. Craniocaudal
    c. Mediolateral oblique
    d. Exaggerated craniocaudal

15. Which projection requires that the central ray be moved to a horizontal position?

    a. Mediolateral
    b. Craniocaudal
    c. Mediolateral oblique
    d. Exaggerated craniocaudal

CHAPTER 25

Central Nervous System

SECTION 1

Anatomy of the Central Nervous System

Instructions: This exercise pertains to the anatomic structures of the central nervous system (CNS). Identify structures, fill in missing words, or provide a short answer for each item.

1. Identify each lettered structure shown in Fig. 25-1.

A. _____

B. _____

C. _____

D. _____

E. _____

F. _____

G. _____

H. _____

2. Identify each lettered structure shown in Fig. 25-2.

A. _____

B. _____

C. _____

D. _____

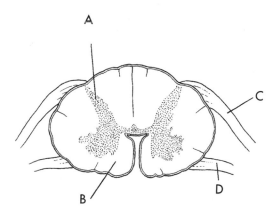

Figure 25-2 Transverse section of the spinal cord.

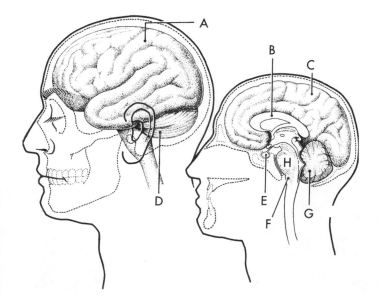

Figure 25-1 Lateral surface and midsection of the brain.

3. Identify each lettered structure shown in Fig. 25-3.

A. _____

B. _____

C. _____

D. _____

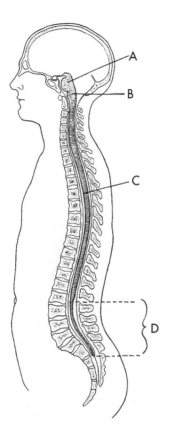

Figure 25-3 Sagittal section showing the spinal cord.

4. Identify each lettered structure shown in Fig. 25-4.

A. _____

B. _____

C. _____

D. _____

E. _____

F. _____

G. _____

H. _____

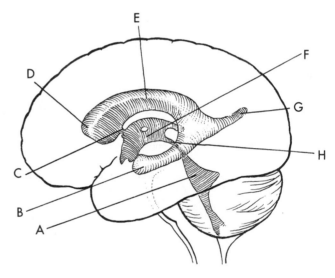

Figure 25-4 Lateral aspect of the cerebral ventricles in relation to the surface of the brain.

5. Identify each lettered structure shown in Fig. 25-5.

A. _____

B. _____

C. _____

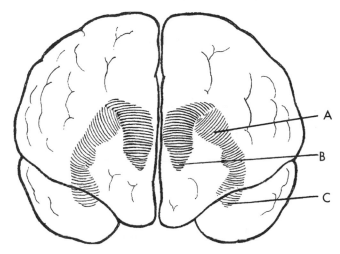

Figure 25-5 Anterior aspect of the lateral cerebral ventricles in relation to the surface of the brain.

6. Identify each lettered structure shown in Fig. 25-6.

A. _____

B. _____

C. _____

D. _____

E. _____

F. _____

G. _____

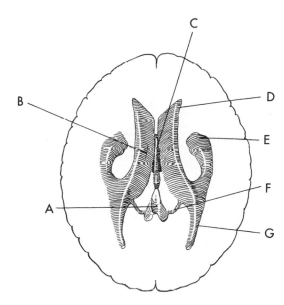

Figure 25-6 Superior aspect of the cerebral ventricles in relation to the surface of the brain.

7. Name the two main parts of the central nervous system.

8. Name the three parts of the brain.

9. Name the four parts of the brain stem.

10. Name the three parts of the hindbrain.

11. The largest part of the brain is the _____.

12. Another name for the cerebrum is the

_____.

13. The stemlike portion of the brain that connects the cerebrum to the hindbrain is the _____.

14. The deep cleft that separates the cerebrum into right and left hemispheres is the _____

_____.

15. Another name for the hypophysis cerebri is

_____ _____.

16. The largest part of the hindbrain is the

_____.

17. The portion of the hindbrain that connects the pons to the spinal cord is the _____

_____.

18. The protective membranes that enclose the brain and spinal cord are the _____.

19. The membrane that closely adheres to the brain and spinal cord is the _____

_____.

20. The outermost membrane that forms the tough fibrous covering for the brain and spinal cord is the

_____ _____.

21. The two uppermost ventricles are called the right and left _____ ventricles.

22. The lateral ventricles are located in the portion of the brain called the _____.

23. Each lateral ventricle communicates with the third ventricle by way of the _____ foramen.

24. Another name for the interventricular foramen is the foramen of _____.

25. What are the two names for the passage between the third and fourth ventricles?

SECTION 2

Radiography of the Central Nervous System

Instructions: This exercise pertains to examinations that demonstrate central nervous system structures. Provide a short answer for each item.

1. Define myelography.

2. Identify three common sites for the injection of the contrast medium during myelography.

3. What abnormality is demonstrated using myelography?

4. What type or group of contrast media is preferred for myelography? Explain why.

5. When the exposure room is prepared for myelography, why should the spot-filming device be locked in place?

6. What should be done to reduce patient apprehension?

7. What are the two body positions most frequently used when the contrast medium is injected for myelography?

8. During myelography, what procedure is used to control the movement of the contrast medium after its injection?

9. During myelography, why should the patient hyperextend the neck?

10. When a traumatized patient with possible CNS involvement is radiographed, what radiograph should be the first one made?

Self-Test: Central Nervous System

Instructions: Answer the following questions by selecting the best choice.

1. Which two structures comprise the CNS?

    a. Brain and cerebellum
    b. Brain and spinal cord
    c. Cerebrum and cerebellum
    d. Cerebrum and spinal cord

2. Which part of the brain is also referred to as the forebrain?

    a. Pons
    b. Cerebrum
    c. Cerebellum
    d. Diencephalon

3. Which three parts of the CNS comprise the hindbrain?

    a. Cerebrum, cerebellum, and spinal cord
    b. Cerebrum, pons, and medulla oblongata
    c. Pons, cerebellum, and medulla oblongata
    d. Pons, spinal cord, and medulla oblongata

4. Which cerebral structure is the largest part of the brain?

    a. Pons
    b. Cerebrum
    c. Cerebellum
    d. Medulla oblongata

5. Which structure is divided into right and left hemispheres by the longitudinal fissure?

    a. Pons
    b. Cerebrum
    c. Cerebellum
    d. Medulla oblongata

6. What other term refers to the hypophysis cerebri?

    a. Pituitary gland
    b. Medulla spinalis
    c. Corpus callosum
    d. Conus medullaris

7. Which membrane forms the tough, fibrous outer covering for the meninges?

    a. Pia mater
    b. Arachnoid
    c. Dura mater

8. Which vessel connects the lateral ventricles to the third ventricle?

    a. Cerebral aqueduct
    b. Foramen of Luschka
    c. Foramen of Magendie
    d. Interventricular foramen

9. In which part of the brain is the fourth ventricle found?

    a. Midbrain
    b. Forebrain
    c. Hindbrain

10. Which projection should be the first radiograph for a traumatized patient with possible CNS involvement?

    a. AP axial
    b. AP oblique
    c. Upright lateral
    d. Cross-table lateral

11. Which examination is performed to demonstrate the contour of the subarachnoid space?

    a. Diskography
    b. Myelography
    c. Ventriculography
    d. Pneumonography

12. For which examination is the contrast medium injected directly into the fibrous cartilage between two vertebral bodies?

    a. Diskography
    b. Myelography
    c. Ventriculography
    d. Pneumonography

13. Which examination can be used to evaluate the dynamic flow pattern of cerebral spinal fluid?

    a. Diskography
    b. Myelography
    c. Ventriculography
    d. Pneumonography

14. During myelography, which procedure should be performed to prevent contrast medium from entering the cerebral ventricles?

    a. Tilt the head of the table down.
    b. Instruct the patient to hyperflex the neck.
    c. Place the patient in the lateral recumbent position.
    d. Have the patient hyperextend the neck.

15. What is the purpose of tilting the table during myelography?

    a. To attach the footboard
    b. To facilitate patient comfort
    c. To control the flow of contrast medium
    d. To remove cerebral spinal fluid from the patient

CHAPTER 26

Circulatory System

SECTION 1

Anatomy of the Circulatory System

Exercise 1

Instructions: This exercise pertains to the anatomy of the circulatory system. Identify structures for each item.

1. Identify each lettered structure shown in Fig. 26-1.

A. _____

B. _____

C. _____

D. _____

E. _____

F. _____

G. _____

H. _____

I. _____

J. _____

K. _____

L. _____

M. _____

N. _____

O. _____

P. _____

Q. _____

R. _____

S. _____

T. _____

U. _____

V. _____

W. _____

X. _____

Y. _____

Z. _____

AA. _____

BB. _____

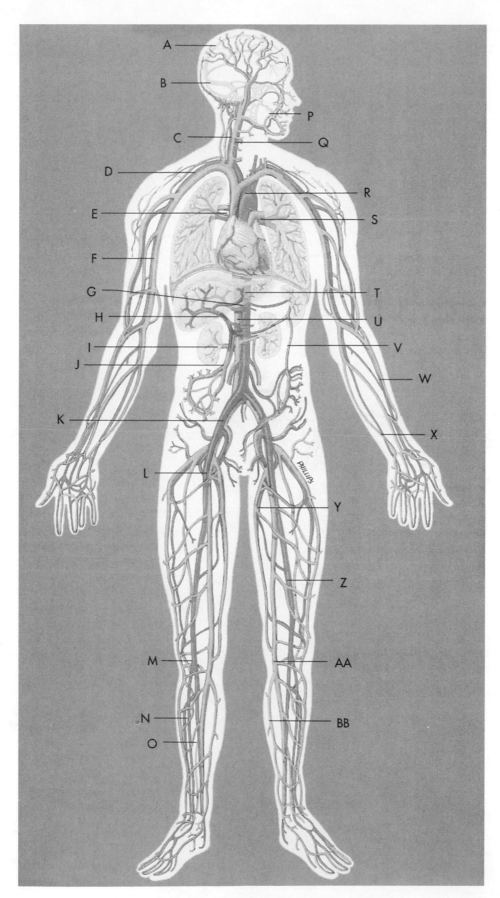

Figure 26-1 Major arteries and veins.

2. Identify each lettered structure shown in Fig. 26-2.

A. _____

B. _____

C. _____

D. _____

E. _____

F. _____

G. _____

H. _____

I. _____

J. _____

K. _____

L. _____

M. _____

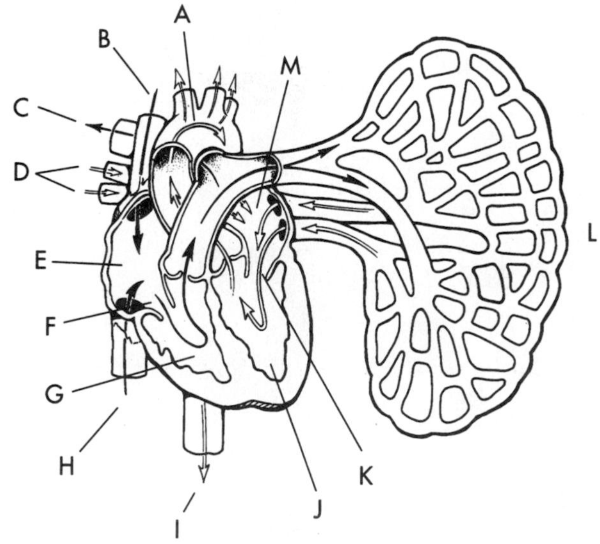

Figure 26-2 The heart and greater vessels. Black arrows indicate deoxygenated blood flow. White arrows indicate oxygenated blood flow.

3. Identify each lettered structure shown in Fig. 26-3.

A. _____

B. _____

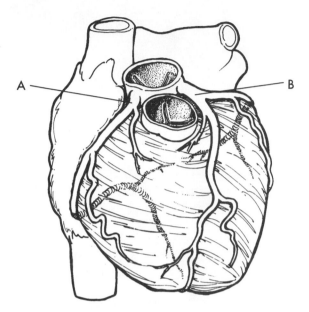

Figure 26-3 Anterior view of the coronary arteries.

4. Identify each lettered structure shown in Fig. 26-4.

A. _____

B. _____

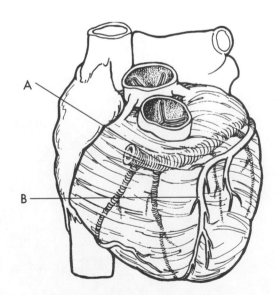

Figure 26-4 Anterior view of the coronary veins.

5. Identify each lettered structure shown in Fig. 26-5.

A. _____

B. _____

C. _____

D. _____

E. _____

F. _____

G. _____

H. _____

I. _____

J. _____

K. _____

L. _____

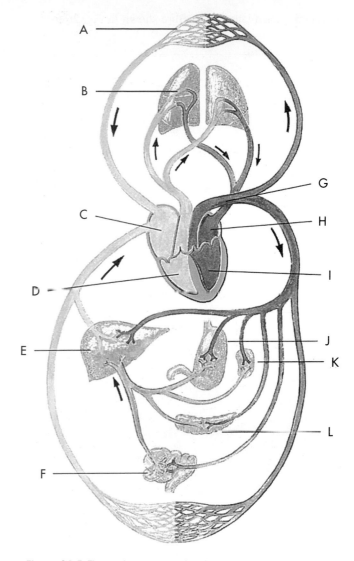

Figure 26-5 The pulmonary, systemic, and portal circulation.

6. Identify each lettered structure shown in Fig. 26-6.

A. _____   H. _____

B. _____   I. _____

C. _____   J. _____

D. _____   K. _____

E. _____   L. _____

F. _____   M. _____

G. _____

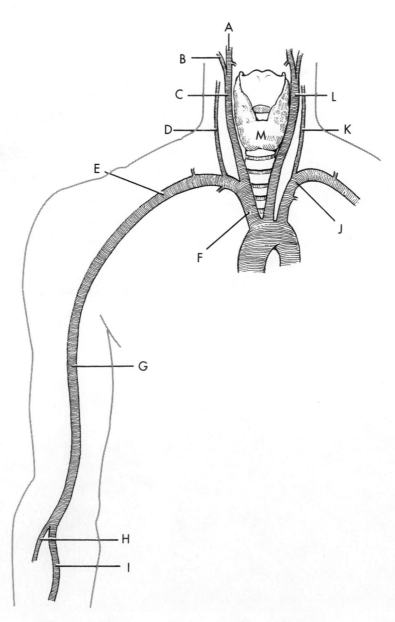

Figure 26-6 Major arteries of the upper chest, neck, and arm.

7. Identify each lettered structure shown in Fig. 26-7.

A. _____   E. _____

B. _____   F. _____

C. _____   G. _____

D. _____

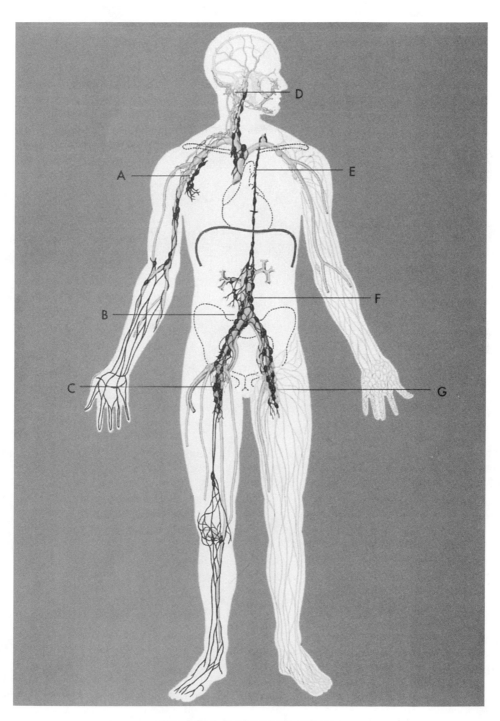

Figure 26-7 The lymphatic system.

Exercise 2

Instructions: This exercise is a comprehensive review of the circulatory system. Fill in missing words for each item.

1. The circulatory system comprises two systems of related vessels, the _____ system and the _____ system.

2. The two systems that comprise the blood-vascular system are _____ circulation and _____ circulation.

3. The system that traverses the lungs to discharge carbon dioxide and take up oxygen is _____ circulation.

4. The vessels that carry blood away from the heart are collectively called _____.

5. The vessels that carry blood back toward the heart are collectively called _____.

6. Arteries subdivide to form _____.

7. Arterioles subdivide to form _____.

8. Capillaries unite to form _____.

9. The beginning branches for veins are _____.

10. Blood is transported to the left atrium by _____ veins.

11. The major vein that returns blood from the upper parts of the body to the heart is the _____ _____.

12. The major vein that returns blood from the lower parts of the body to the heart is the _____ _____.

13. The muscular wall of the heart is the _____.

14. The membrane that lines the chambers of the heart is the _____.

15. The membrane that covers the heart is the _____.

16. The chamber of the heart where the myocardium is the thickest is the _____ _____.

17. The space between the two walls of the pericardial sac is the _____ _____.

18. The two upper chambers of the heart are the _____.

19. The two lower chambers of the heart are the _____.

20. The receiving chambers of the heart are the _____.

21. The distributing chambers of the heart are the _____.

22. Another name for the right atrioventricular valve is the _____ valve.

23. Two other terms that refer to the left atrioventricular valve are the _____ valve and the _____ valve.

24. The side of the heart that pumps venous (deoxygenated) blood is the _____ (right or left) side.

25. The side of the heart that pumps arterial (oxygenated) blood is the _____ (right or left) side.

26. The chamber of the heart that pumps blood through the aortic valve is the _____ _____.

27. The vessels that supply blood to the myocardium are the right and left _____ arteries.

28. The coronary sinus receives blood from the _____ veins.

29. The coronary sinus empties blood into the _____ (right or left) atrium.

30. The great vessel that arises from the left ventricle to transport blood to the body is the _____.

31. The abdominal aorta divides into the right and left common _____ arteries.

32. The external iliac artery enters the lower limb and becomes the _____ artery.

33. The femoral artery passes blood into the _____ artery.

34. The popliteal artery bifurcates into the anterior and posterior _____ arteries.

35. The vessel that drains blood into the liver is the _____ vein.

36. The vessels that drain blood from the liver are the _____ veins.

37. Hepatic veins transport blood to the _____ _____ _____.

38. The large vessel that arises from the right atrium is the _____ artery.

39. The only arteries of the body that transport deoxygenated blood are the _____ arteries.

40. The only veins of the body that transport oxygenated blood are the _____ veins.

41. The contraction phase of the heart is called the _____.

42. The relaxation phase of the heart is called the _____.

43. The four arteries that supply the brain are the right and left _____ _____ arteries and the right and left _____ arteries.

44. Of the four trunk arteries that supply the brain, the one that arises directly from the arch of the aorta is the _____ _____ _____ artery.

45. The right and left vertebral arteries arise from the _____ arteries.

46. The right and left vertebral arteries unite to form the _____ artery.

47. Each common carotid artery bifurcates into the _____ and _____ carotid arteries.

48. Each internal carotid artery bifurcates into anterior and middle _____ arteries.

49. The basilar artery bifurcates into the right and left _____ _____ arteries.

50. Blood is drained from the head by the

_____ veins.

51. To reach the right subclavian artery, blood passes from the

aorta through the _____ artery.

52. Blood passes from the brachiocephalic artery to the right

_____ artery.

53. A subclavian artery supplies blood to the axillary artery

and then to the _____ artery.

54. The brachial arteries bifurcate into the

_____ and

_____ arteries.

55. The part of the body in which the cephalic vein originates

is the _____.

56. The renal arteries arise from the

_____.

57. The circle of Willis is located within the

_____.

58. The central organ of the blood–vascular system is the

_____.

59. The main terminal trunk of the lymphatic system is the

_____ duct.

60. The thoracic duct drains its contents at the junction of the

left _____ vein and the internal

_____ vein.

SECTION 2

Radiography of the Circulatory System

Instructions: This exercise pertains to various radiographic examinations for the circulatory system. Because many of these procedures are dependent on the preferences of the radiologist, most of the following exercise items are general in content rather than emphasizing a specific procedure. Identify structures, fill in missing words, select from a list, or provide a short answer for each item.

1. List four reasons that catheterization is preferred over direct injection of the contrast medium through a needle.

2. The most widely used method of catheterization is the

   _____ technique.

3. The preferred site for insertion of the catheter for most selective angiography is the _____ artery.

4. What is the purpose of side holes near the tip of the catheter?

   a. To draw fluid into the catheter
   b. To reduce whiplash, stabilizing the catheter
   c. To maintain positive pressure inside the catheter

5. From the following list, circle the three symptoms of a vasovagal reaction that are caused by the injection of the contrast medium.

   a. Hives
   b. Nausea
   c. Sweating
   d. Difficult breathing
   e. Increase in pulse rate
   f. Increase in blood pressure
   g. Decrease in blood pressure

6. From the following list, circle the three symptoms of shock.

   a. Low pulse rate
   b. High pulse rate
   c. Rapid breathing
   d. Shallow breathing
   e. Loss of consciousness
   f. Rise in body temperature

7. What treatment should be given to patients experiencing low blood pressure because of a vasovagal reaction?

8. In preparation for angiography, why should the patient be instructed not to consume solid food?

9. In preparation for angiography, why should the patient be allowed to drink clear liquids?

10. For thoracic aortography, to which vertebra should the perpendicular central ray be directed?

11. Identify each lettered structure shown in Fig. 26-8.

A. _____ E. _____

B. _____ F. _____

C. _____ G. _____

D. _____ H. _____

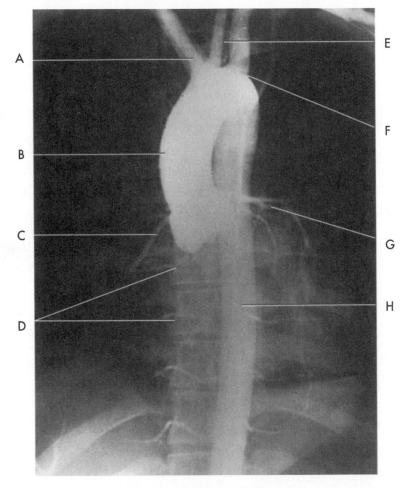

Figure 26-8 AP thoracic aortogram.

12. How much of the aorta should be imaged for abdominal aortography?

13. For abdominal aortography, which projection of the abdominal aorta—anteroposterior (AP) or lateral—best demonstrates the celiac and superior mesenteric artery origins?

14. Identify each lettered structure shown in Fig. 26-9.

    A. _____

    B. _____

    C. _____

    D. _____

    E. _____

    F. _____

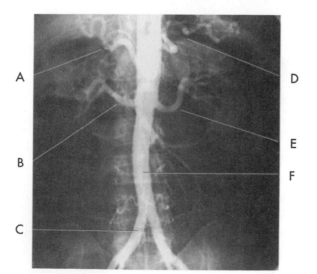

Figure 26-9 AP abdominal aortogram.

15. Identify each lettered structure shown in Fig. 26-10.

    A. _____

    B. _____

    C. _____

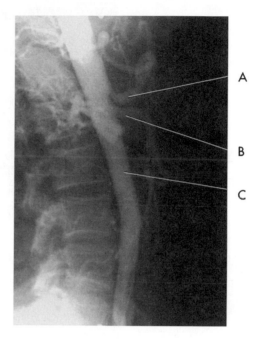

Figure 26-10 Lateral abdominal aortogram.

16. For pulmonary arteriography, which projection—AP or lateral—should use a compensating (trough) filter to obtain a radiograph with more uniform density between the vertebrae and the lungs?

    _____

17. All radiographs for selective abdominal visceral arteriography should be exposed when the patient has suspended

    _____ (inspiration or expiration).

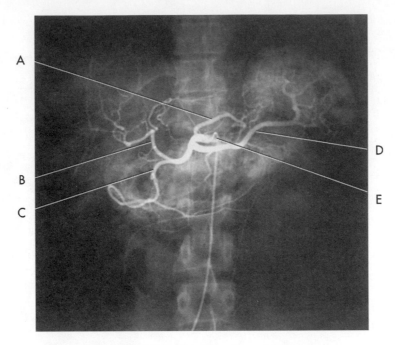

Figure 26-11 Selective AP celiac arteriogram.

18. Identify each lettered structure shown in Fig. 26-11.

   A. _____

   B. _____

   C. _____

   D. _____

   E. _____

19. What is the advantage of examining the patient's intravenous urography radiographs before positioning the patient for a renal arteriogram?

20. For demonstrating the portal venous system, the contrast medium should be injected into the

   _____ artery.

21. Blood in veins flows _____ (proximally or distally).

22. For renal venography, the renal vein is most easily catheterized using the _____ (upper or lower) limb approach.

23. Into which vein should a catheter be positioned to best demonstrate the superior vena cava?

   a. Subclavian
   b. Common iliac
   c. Inferior vena cava

24. Into which vein should a catheter be positioned to best demonstrate the inferior vena cava?

   a. Portal
   b. Common iliac
   c. Superior vena cava

25. Into which artery should the catheter be positioned to best demonstrate the arteries of an entire upper limb with a single injection of contrast medium?

   a. Femoral
   b. Subclavian
   c. Common iliac

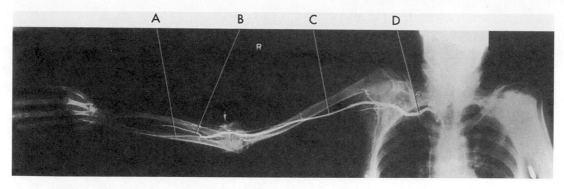

Figure 26-12 Right upper-limb arteriogram. (The radial artery is not demonstrated due to occlusion.)

26. Identify each lettered structure shown in Fig. 26-12.

A. _____

B. _____

C. _____

D. _____

27. Where is the injection site for the introduction of contrast medium for upperlimb venography?

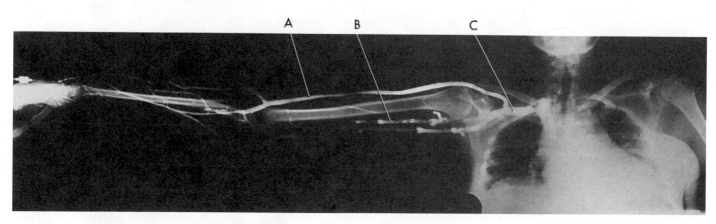

Figure 26-13 Right upper-limb venogram.

28. Identify each lettered structure shown in Fig. 26-13.

A. _____

B. _____

C. _____

29. For simultaneous bilateral femoral arteriograms, how should the patient's legs be positioned?

30. Identify each lettered structure shown in Fig. 26-14.

A. _____

B. _____

C. _____

D. _____

E. _____

F. _____

G. _____

H. _____

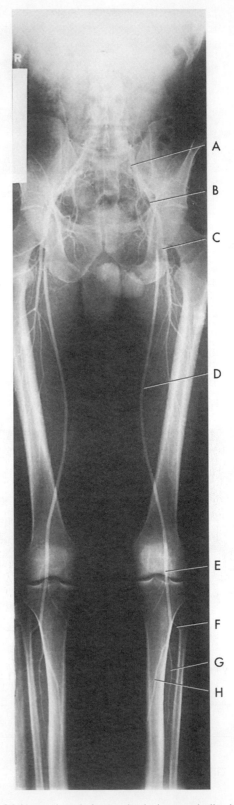

Figure 26-14 Normal aortofemoral arteriogram in the late arterial phase.

31. At what area of the leg should radiographs begin for lowerlimb venography?

    a. Hip
    b. Knee
    c. Ankle

32. For lowerlimb venography, what is the purpose of applying tourniquets just proximal to the ankle and knee?

    a. To stop the pulse within the leg
    b. To prevent blood flow into the leg
    c. To force the filling of the deep veins of the leg

33. Approximately how many seconds does it take for blood to flow from the internal carotid artery to the jugular vein in cerebral angiography?

    a. 3 seconds
    b. 6 seconds
    c. 9 seconds

34. Why should the first radiograph of a cerebral arteriography series be made before the arrival of the contrast medium?

    a. To check exposure factors
    b. To confirm patient positioning
    c. To serve as a subtraction mask
    d. To demonstrate soft-tissue abnormalities

35. What is the visualization sequence for the three phases of blood flow that should be seen in cerebral angiography?

    a. Arterial, capillary, and venous
    b. Arterial, venous, and capillary
    c. Capillary, arterial, and venous
    d. Capillary, venous, and arterial
    e. Venous, arterial, and capillary
    f. Venous, capillary, and arterial

36. Figs. 26-15, 26-16, and 26-17 are cerebral angiograms, and each shows a phase of blood flow. Examine each image and identify which phase of blood flow—arterial, capillary, or venous—the image represents.

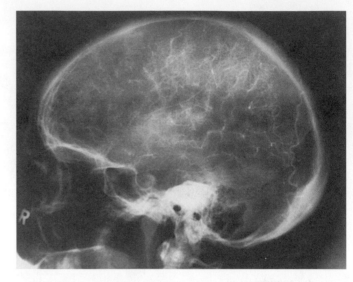

Figure 26-15 Cerebral angiogram.

a. Figure 26-15: _____

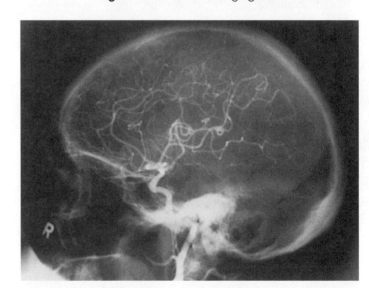

Figure 26-16 Cerebral angiogram.

b. Figure 26-16: _____

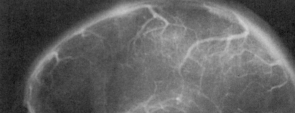

Figure 26-17 Cerebral angiogram.

c. Figure 26-17: _____

37. For the basic AP projection during cerebral angiography, what positioning line of the skull should be perpendicular to the horizontal plane?

38. For the AP axial oblique projection (transorbital) demonstrating anterior circulation during cerebral angiography, in which direction—toward the injected side or away from the injected side—should the head be rotated?

39. For the AP axial projection (supraorbital) demonstrating anterior circulation during cerebral angiography, how should the central ray be directed to project the vessels above the floor of the anterior cranial fossa?
    a. Caudally
    b. Cephalically
    c. Perpendicularly

40. For the AP axial oblique projection (transorbital) demonstrating the internal carotid bifurcation and the anterior communicating and middle cerebral arteries within the orbital shadow, how should the central ray be directed?
    a. Caudally
    b. Cephalically
    c. Perpendicularly

Self-Test: Anatomy and Radiography of the Circulatory System

Instructions: Answer the following questions by selecting the best choice.

1. Which vessels originate immediately because of the division of arteries?
   a. Veins
   b. Venules
   c. Arterioles
   d. Capillaries

2. In which part of the body is the basilic vein located?
   a. Head
   b. Abdomen
   c. Lower limb
   d. Upper limb

3. Which chamber of the heart receives deoxygenated blood?
   a. Left atrium
   b. Left ventricle
   c. Right atrium
   d. Right ventricle

4. Which chamber of the heart receives blood from the pulmonary veins?
   a. Left atrium
   b. Left ventricle
   c. Right atrium
   d. Right ventricle

5. What is the purpose of the septa of the heart?
   a. To separate atria from ventricles
   b. To provide openings into the atria
   c. To form the atrioventricular valves
   d. To divide the heart into right and left halves

6. The circuit for blood flow from the left ventricle to the right atrium is _____ circulation.
   a. deep
   b. systemic
   c. superficial
   d. pulmonary

7. Which arteries are the first to branch from the ascending aorta?
   a. Coronary
   b. Vertebral
   c. Subclavian
   d. Common carotid

8. Through which valve does blood pass when it exits the heart for systemic circulation?
   a. Aortic
   b. Mitral
   c. Bicuspid
   d. Tricuspid

9. Which of the following is a disadvantage of nonionic contrast agents compared with ionic contrast agents of lower iodine concentrations?
   a. Increased viscosity
   b. Increased cardiovascular side effects
   c. Increased exposure factor requirements
   d. Decreased radiographic contrast of opacified vessels

10. Why can exposures not occur in both planes at the same moment during simultaneous biplane imaging?
    a. X-ray tubes will overload.
    b. Scatter radiation will fog the images.
    c. Two injections of contrast medium are required.
    d. X-ray generators cannot be synchronized for multiple exposures.

11. Which procedure should be performed to reduce the magnification of structures for lateral projections during thoracic aortography?
    a. Use an image receptor (IR) changer.
    b. Use the smallest available focal spot.
    c. Increase the source-to-IR distance (SID).
    d. Increase the object-to-IR distance (OID).

12. Which arteriogram requires the use of a compensating (trough) filter to obtain a more uniform density between the vertebral structures and lungs?
    a. AP celiac axis
    b. AP pulmonary
    c. Lateral pulmonary
    d. AP superior mesenteric

13. To which level of the patient should the IR and central ray be centered for AP abdominal aortograms?
    a. T6
    b. T10
    c. L2
    d. Iliac crests

14. To which level of the patient should the IR and central ray be centered for celiac arteriograms?
    a. T2
    b. T6
    c. L2
    d. S1

15. Which area of the patient should be prepared for the injection of contrast medium for cephalic venography?

    a. Thigh
    b. Ankle
    c. Wrist
    d. Upper arm

16. Which area of the patient should be prepared for the injection of contrast medium for demonstration of the superior vena cava?

    a. Thigh
    b. Ankle
    c. Wrist
    d. Upper arm

17. Which area of the patient is the preferred site for insertion of the catheter through the skin for internal carotid arteriography?

    a. Neck
    b. Thigh
    c. Abdomen
    d. Upper arm

18. Why should a radiograph be taken before the arrival of contrast medium for cerebral angiography?

    a. To serve as a subtraction mask
    b. To ensure that collimation is adequate
    c. To check for proper positioning of the patient
    d. To verify that the correct exposure factors are used

19. Which phase of blood flow should have the most films exposed during cerebral angiography?

    a. Venous
    b. Arterial
    c. Capillary
    d. Parenchymal

20. Which positioning line of the skull should be perpendicular to the horizontal plane for basic AP projections during cerebral arteriography?

    a. Orbitomeatal
    b. Glabellomeatal
    c. Acanthiomeatal
    d. Infraorbitomeatal

CHAPTER 27

Sectional Anatomy for Radiographers

Review

Instructions: It is essential that the radiographer have an understanding of the relationships between organ and skeletal structures to perform computed tomography (CT), magnetic resonance imaging (MRI), and diagnostic ultrasound examinations because all three modalities create images of sectional anatomy. This exercise is a review of sectional anatomy. Identify structures for each item.

Fig. 27-1 shows a CT localizer, or scout, image of the skull. Figs. 27-2 through 27-5 pertain to the imaging planes shown in Fig. 27-1.

1. Identify each lettered structure shown in Fig. 27-2.

   A. _____

   B. _____

   C. _____

   D. _____

   E. _____

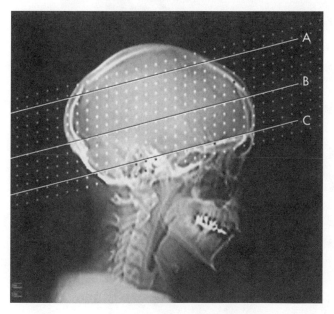

Figure 27-1 CT localizer, or scout, image of the skull.

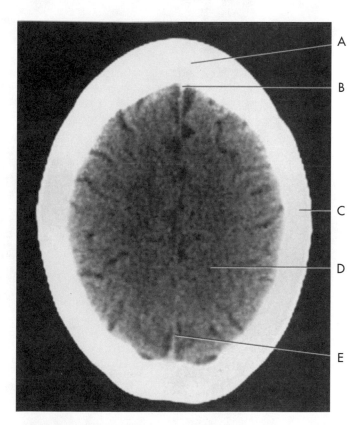

Figure 27-2 CT image corresponding to level A in Fig. 27-1.

239

2. Identify each lettered structure shown in Fig. 27-3.

A. _____   F. _____

B. _____   G. _____

C. _____   H. _____

D. _____   I. _____

E. _____   J. _____

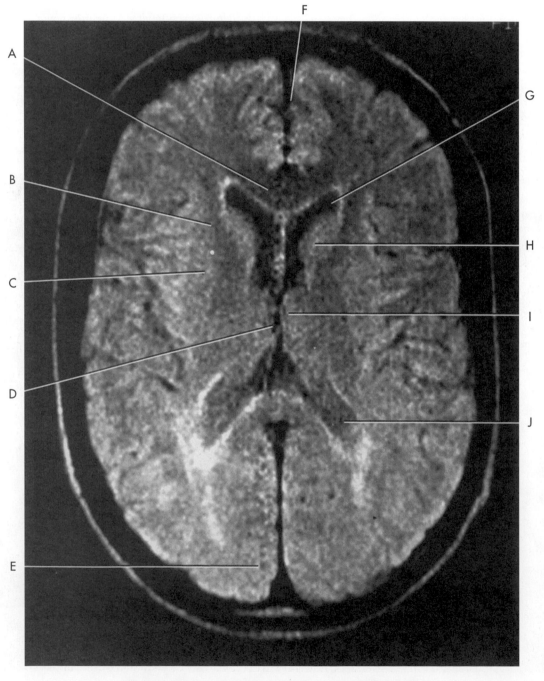

Figure 27-3 MRI image corresponding to level B in Fig. 27-1.

3. Identify each lettered structure shown in Fig. 27-4.

A. _____

B. _____

C. _____

D. _____

E. _____

F. _____

G. _____

H. _____

I. _____

J. _____

K. _____

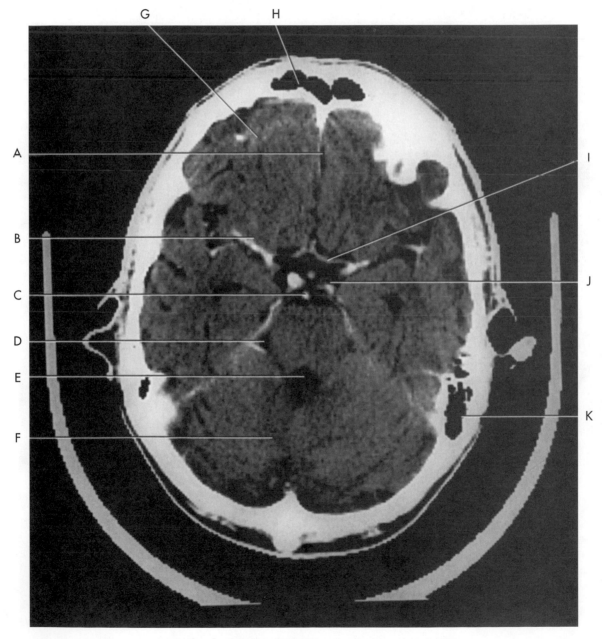

Figure 27-4 CT image corresponding to level C in Fig. 27-1.

4. Identify each lettered structure shown in Fig. 27-5.

A. _____   G. _____

B. _____   H. _____

C. _____   I. _____

D. _____   J. _____

E. _____   K. _____

F. _____

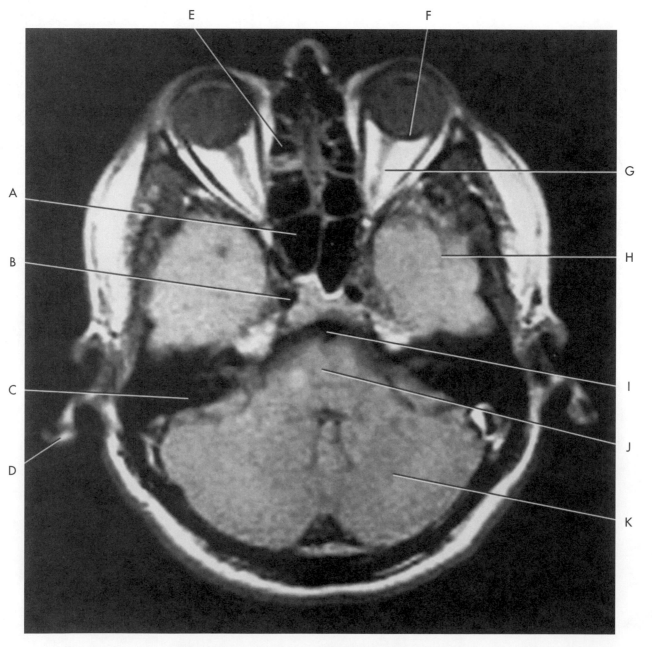

Figure 27-5 MRI image corresponding to level C in Fig. 27-1.

5. Identify each lettered structure shown in Fig. 27-6.

A. _____

B. _____

C. _____

D. _____

E. _____

F. _____

G. _____

H. _____

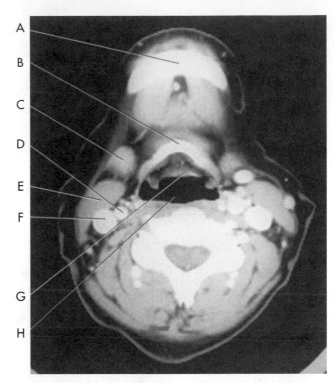

Figure 27-6 CT image through the fourth cervical vertebra.

6. Identify each lettered structure shown in Fig. 27-7.

A. _____   F. _____

B. _____   G. _____

C. _____   H. _____

D. _____   I. _____

E. _____

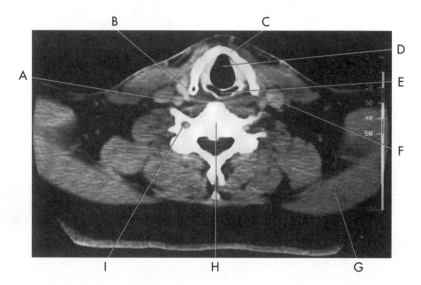

Figure 27-7 CT image through the sixth cervical vertebra.

7. Identify each lettered structure shown in Fig. 27-8.

A. _____

B. _____

C. _____

D. _____

E. _____

F. _____

G. _____

H. _____

I. _____

J. _____

K. _____

L. _____

M. _____

N. _____

O. _____

P. _____

Q. _____

R. _____

S. _____

T. _____

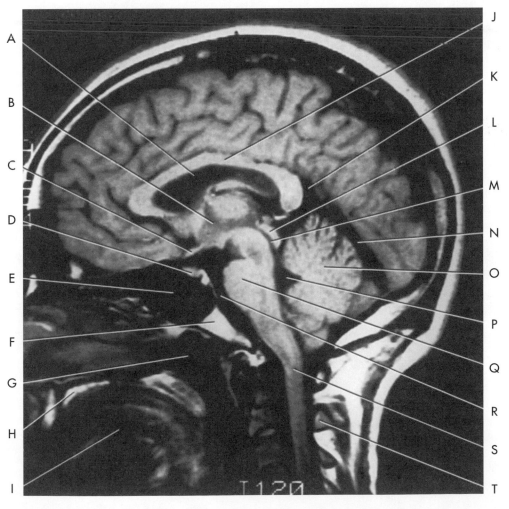

Figure 27-8 Sagittal MRI image through the medial sagittal plane.

Fig. 27-9 shows a CT localizer, or scout, image of the skull. Figs. 27-10, 27-11, and 27-12 pertain to the imaging planes shown in Fig. 27-9.

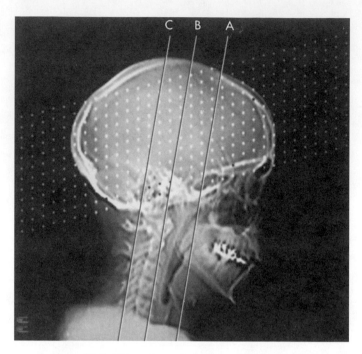

Figure 27-9 CT localizer, or scout, image of the skull.

8. Identify each lettered structure shown in Fig. 27-10.

A. _____

B. _____

C. _____

D. _____

E. _____

F. _____

G. _____

H. _____

I. _____

J. _____

K. _____

L. _____

M. _____

N. _____

O. _____

P. _____

Q. _____

R. _____

S. _____

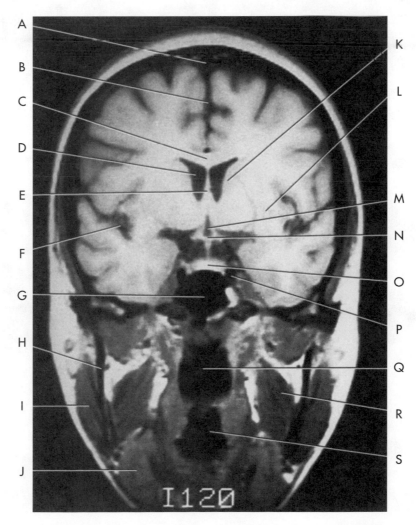

Figure 27-10 Coronal MRI image corresponding to level A in Fig. 27-9.

9. Identify each lettered structure shown in Fig. 27-11.

A. _____   G. _____

B. _____   H. _____

C. _____   I. _____

D. _____   J. _____

E. _____   K. _____

F. _____

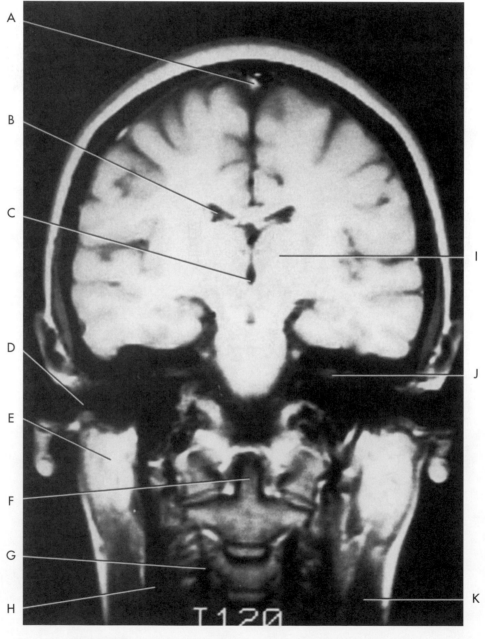

Figure 27-11 Coronal MRI image corresponding to level B in Fig. 27-9.

10. Identify each lettered structure shown in Fig. 27-12.

A. _____

B. _____

C. _____

D. _____

E. _____

F. _____

G. _____

H. _____

I. _____

J. _____

K. _____

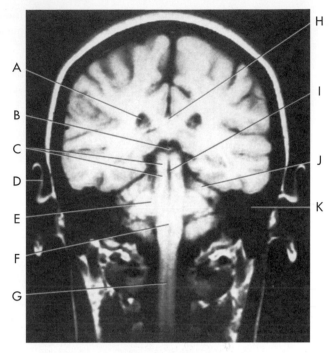

Figure 27-12 Coronal MRI image corresponding to level C in Fig. 27-9.

Fig. 27-13 shows a CT localizer, or scout, image of the thorax. Figs. 27-14, 27-15, and 27-16 pertain to the imaging planes shown in Fig. 27-13.

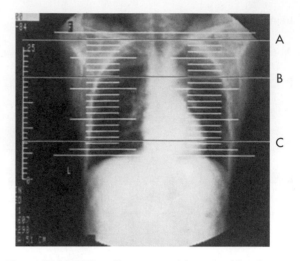

Figure 27-13 CT localizer, or scout, image of the thorax.

11. Identify each lettered structure shown in Fig. 27-14.

A. _____

B. _____

C. _____

D. _____

E. _____

F. _____

G. _____

H. _____

I. _____

J. _____

12. Identify each lettered structure shown in Fig. 27-15.

A. _____

B. _____

C. _____

D. _____

E. _____

F. _____

G. _____

H. _____

I. _____

J. _____

K. _____

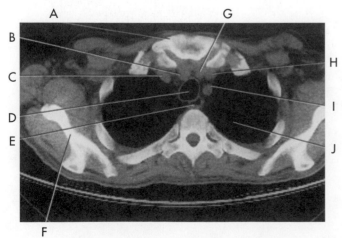

Figure 27-14 CT image corresponding to level A at the second thoracic vertebra in Fig. 27-13.

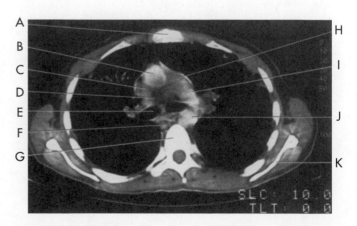

Figure 27-15 CT image corresponding to level B at the fifth thoracic vertebra in Fig. 27-13.

13. Identify each lettered structure shown in Fig. 27-16.

A. _____

B. _____

C. _____

D. _____

E. _____

F. _____

G. _____

H. _____

I. _____

J. _____

K. _____

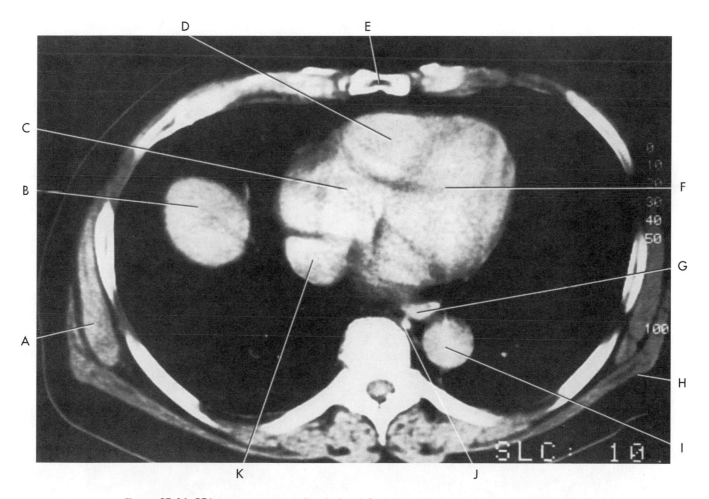

Figure 27-16 CT image corresponding to level C at the ninth thoracic vertebra in Fig. 27-13.

14. Identify each lettered structure shown in Fig. 27-17.

A. _____

B. _____

C. _____

D. _____

E. _____

F. _____

G. _____

H. _____

I. _____

J. _____

K. _____

L. _____

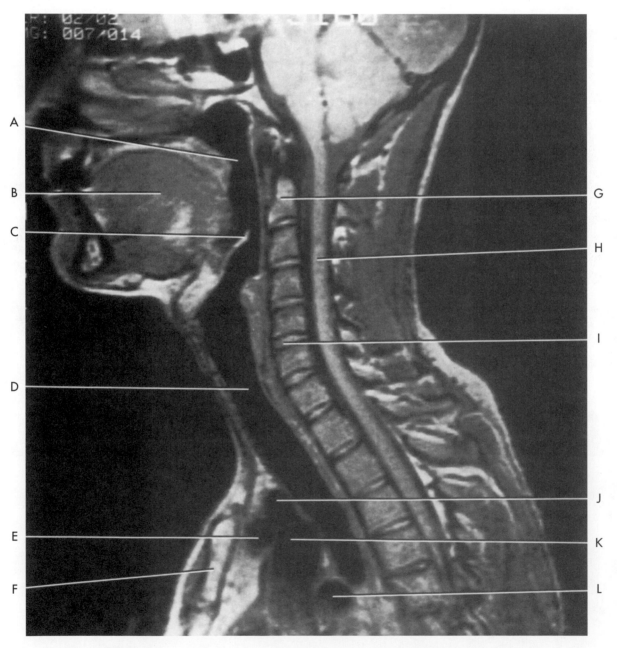

Figure 27-17 Median sagittal MRI image through the neck and upper thorax.

15. Identify each lettered structure shown in Fig. 27-18.

A. _____

B. _____

C. _____

D. _____

E. _____

F. _____

G. _____

H. _____

I. _____

J. _____

K. _____

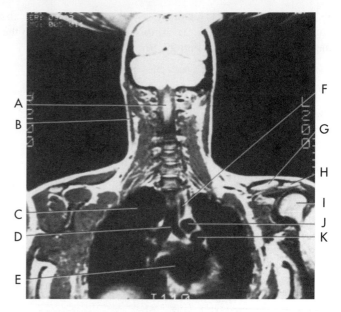

Figure 27-18 MRI image of the neck and thorax through the median coronal plane.

Fig. 27-19 shows a CT localizer, or scout, image of the abdominopelvic region. Figs. 27-20 through 27-26 pertain to the imaging planes shown in Fig. 27-19.

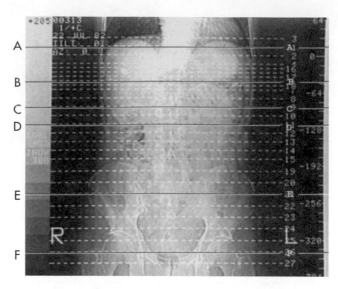

Figure 27-19 CT localizer, or scout, image of the abdominopelvic region.

16. Identify each lettered structure shown in Fig. 27-20.

A. _____

B. _____

C. _____

D. _____

E. _____

F. _____

G. _____

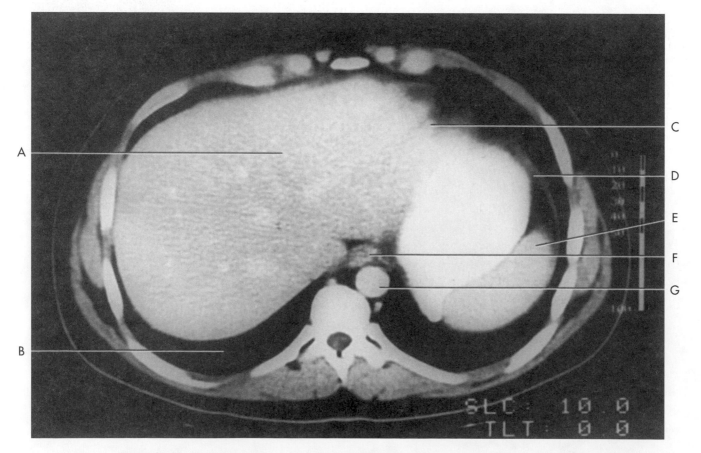

Figure 27-20 CT image corresponding to level A at the 10th thoracic vertebra in Fig. 27-19.

17. Identify each lettered structure shown in Fig. 27-21.

A. _____

B. _____

C. _____

D. _____

E. _____

F. _____

G. _____

H. _____

I. _____

J. _____

K. _____

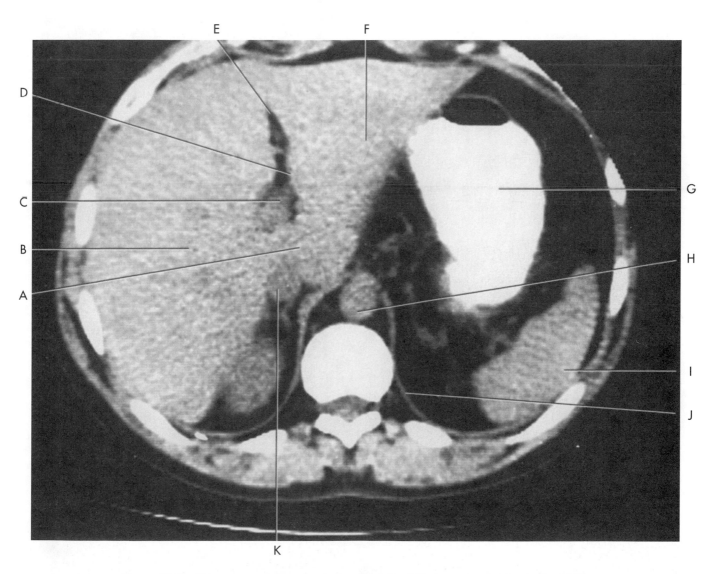

Figure 27-21 CT image corresponding to level B at the 12th thoracic vertebra in Fig. 27-19.

18. Identify each lettered structure shown in Fig. 27-22.

A. _____

B. _____

C. _____

D. _____

E. _____

F. _____

G. _____

H. _____

I. _____

J. _____

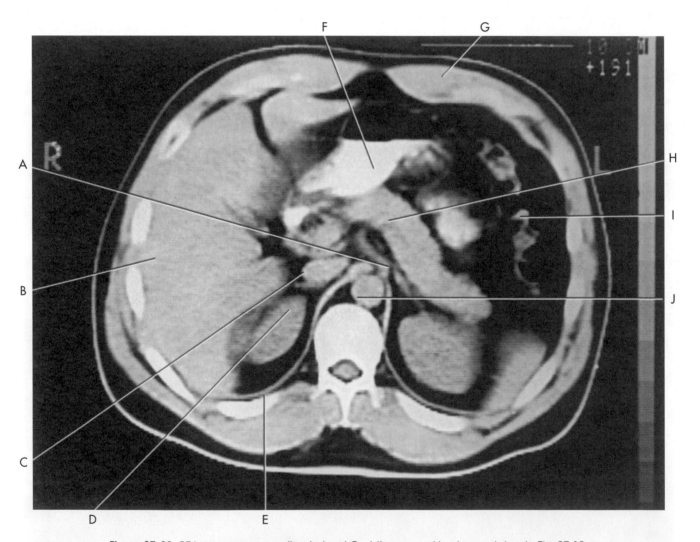

Figure 27-22 CT image corresponding to level C at the second lumbar vertebra in Fig. 27-19.

19. Identify each lettered structure shown in Fig. 27-23.

A. _____

B. _____

C. _____

D. _____

E. _____

F. _____

G. _____

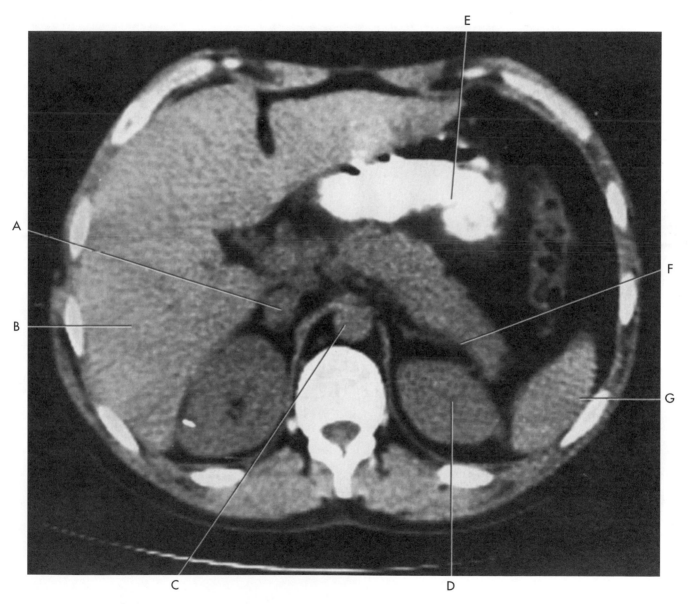

Figure 27-23 CT image corresponding to level D at the interspace between the second and third lumbar vertebrae in Fig. 27-19.

20. Identify each lettered structure shown in Fig. 27-24.

A. _____   E. _____

B. _____   F. _____

C. _____   G. _____

D. _____

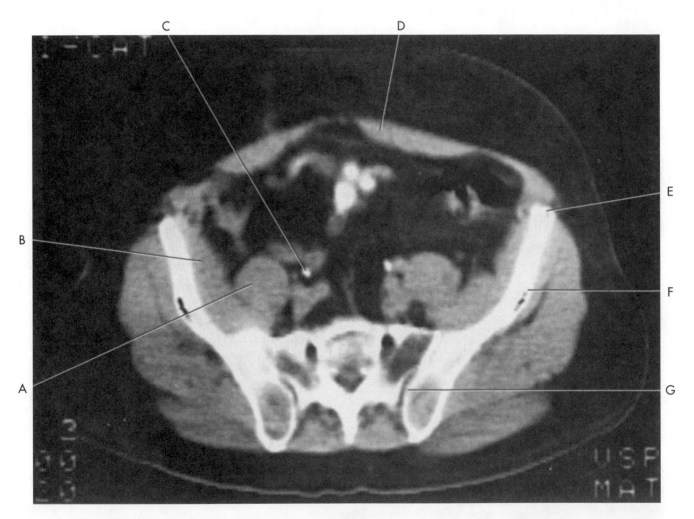

Figure 27-24 CT image corresponding to level E at the anterior superior iliac spine (ASIS) in Fig. 27-19.

21. Identify each lettered structure shown in Fig. 27-25.

A. _____   E. _____

B. _____   F. _____

C. _____   G. _____

D. _____

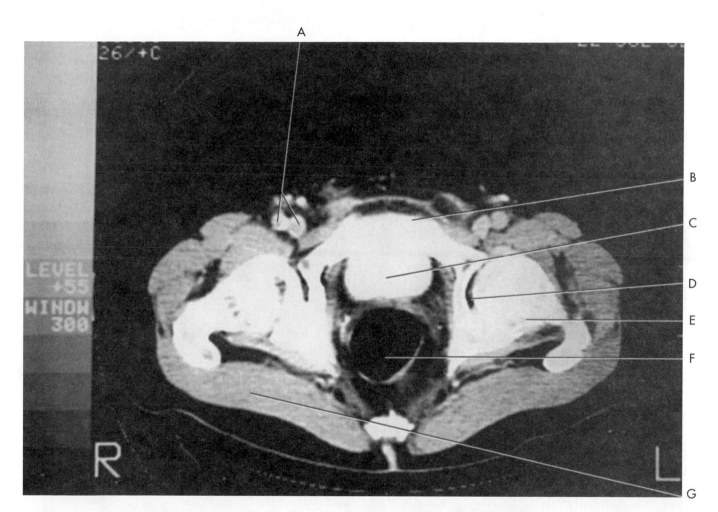

Figure 27-25 CT image corresponding to level F at the coccyx (female) in Fig. 27-19.

22. Identify each lettered structure shown in Fig. 27-26.

A. _____

B. _____

C. _____

D. _____

E. _____

F. _____

G. _____

H. _____

I. _____

J. _____

K. _____

L. _____

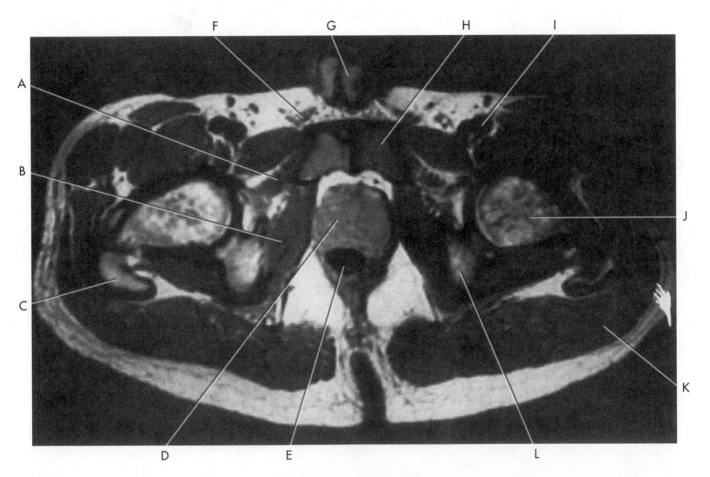

Figure 27-26 CT image corresponding to level F at the coccyx (male) in Fig. 27-19.

23. Identify each lettered structure shown in Fig. 27-27.

A. _____   H. _____

B. _____   I. _____

C. _____   J. _____

D. _____   K. _____

E. _____   L. _____

F. _____   M. _____

G. _____

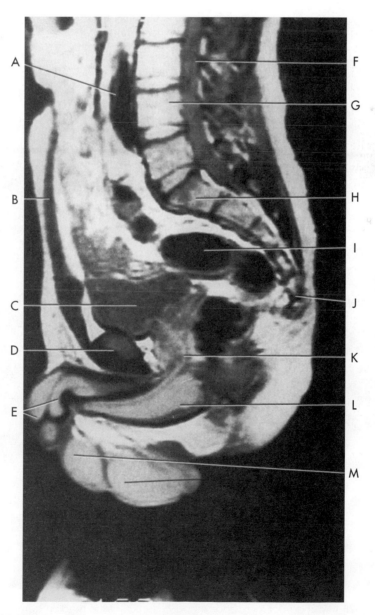

Figure 27-27 MRI image of the abdominopelvic region at the median sagittal plane.

24. Identify each lettered structure shown in Fig. 27-28.

A. _____

B. _____

C. _____

D. _____

E. _____

F. _____

G. _____

H. _____

I. _____

J. _____

K. _____

L. _____

M. _____

N. _____

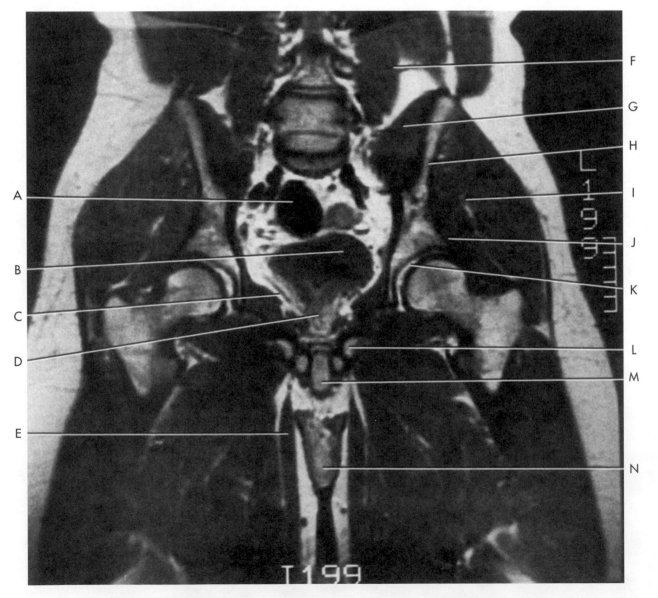

Figure 27-28 MRI image of the abdominopelvic region at the median coronal plane.

Supplemental Exercises for Skull Positioning

Skull Positioning Review

Note to Students: The exercises in this appendix pertain to information referenced from Chapters 20 through 23 and should be completed after you have completed the review exercises for those four chapters.

Exercise 1

Instructions: Match each projection in Column A with the number of degrees and direction of central ray angulation in Column B. Choices from Column B may be used once, more than once, or not at all.

Column A

_____ 1. AP axial (facial bones)

_____ 2. AP axial (cranium; Towne method)

_____ 3. AP axial (temporomandibular articulations)

_____ 4. AP axial (zygomatic arches; modified Towne method)

_____ 5. PA (sphenoidal sinuses)

_____ 6. PA axial (cranium; Haas method)

_____ 7. PA axial (sinuses; Caldwell method)

_____ 8. PA axial (cranium; Caldwell method)

_____ 9. Axiolateral oblique (mandible)

_____ 10. Axiolateral oblique (temporomandibular articulations)

_____ 11. Axiolateral oblique (petromastoid portion; Arcelin method [anterior profile])

_____ 12. Axiolateral oblique (petromastoid portion; Stenvers method [posterior profile])

_____ 13. Parietoacanthial (sinuses; Waters method)

_____ 14. Parieto-orbital oblique (optic foramen; Rhese method)

_____ 15. Axiolateral (mastoids; modified Law method [single-tube angulation method])

Column B

a. Perpendicular

b. 10 degrees caudad

c. 10 degrees cephalad

d. 12 degrees caudad

e. 12 degrees cephalad

f. 15 degrees caudad

g. 15 degrees cephalad

h. 20 degrees caudad

i. 20 degrees cephalad

j. 23 degrees caudad

k. 23 degrees cephalad

l. 25 degrees caudad

m. 25 degrees cephalad

n. 30 degrees caudad

o. 30 degrees cephalad

p. 35 degrees caudad

q. 35 degrees cephalad

r. 37 degrees cephalad

Exercise 2

Instructions: Match the projections in Column A with the locations in Column B. Each location in Column B is either a centering point for the body part or a point where the central ray should enter or exit the patient. Not all locations in Column B may apply to the projections listed in Column B.

Column A

_____ 1. Lateral (cranium)

_____ 2. Lateral (nasal bones)

_____ 3. Lateral (facial bones)

_____ 4. Lateral (sella turcica)

_____ 5. Lateral (paranasal sinuses)

_____ 6. Tangential (zygomatic arch)

_____ 7. PA axial (cranium; Haas method)

_____ 8. PA axial (cranium; Caldwell method)

_____ 9. Parietoacanthial (sinuses; Waters method)

_____ 10. AP axial (zygomatic arches)

_____ 11. AP axial (temporomandibular articulations)

_____ 12. Axiolateral oblique (temporomandibular articulations)

_____ 13. Axiolateral oblique (petromastoid portion; Arcelin method [anterior profile])

_____ 14. Axiolateral oblique (petromastoid portion; Stenvers method [posterior profile])

_____ 15. Axiolateral (mastoids; modified Law method [single-tube angulation method])

Column B

a. Nasion

b. Glabella

c. Acanthion

d. Zygomatic bone

e. External acoustic meatus (EAM)

f. $\frac{1}{2}$ inch (1.2 cm) distal to the nasion

g. $1\frac{1}{2}$ inches (3.8 cm) above the nasion

h. 3 inches (7.6 cm) above the nasion

i. $\frac{1}{2}$ to 1 inch (1.2 to 2.5 cm) posterior to the outer canthus

j. $1\frac{1}{2}$ inches (3.8 cm) posterior to the outer canthus

k. $\frac{1}{2}$ inch (1.2 cm) anterior to the EAM

l. 1 inch (2.5 cm) anterior to the EAM

m. 1 inch (2.5 cm) posterior to the EAM

n. 2 inches (5 cm) superior to the EAM

o. $\frac{3}{4}$ inch (1.9 cm) anterior and $\frac{3}{4}$ inch (1.9 cm) superior to the EAM

p. 1 inch (2.5 cm) anterior and $\frac{3}{4}$ inch (1.9 cm) superior to the EAM

Exercise 3

Instructions: Examine the following diagrams of various projections of the skull (e.g., cranium, facial bones, sinuses). Listed after the diagrams are the names and characteristics of skull projections. In the space provided, write the letter of the diagram that corresponds to each name or characteristic. Not all diagrams may apply to the listed names and characteristics, and some diagrams may be used more than once.

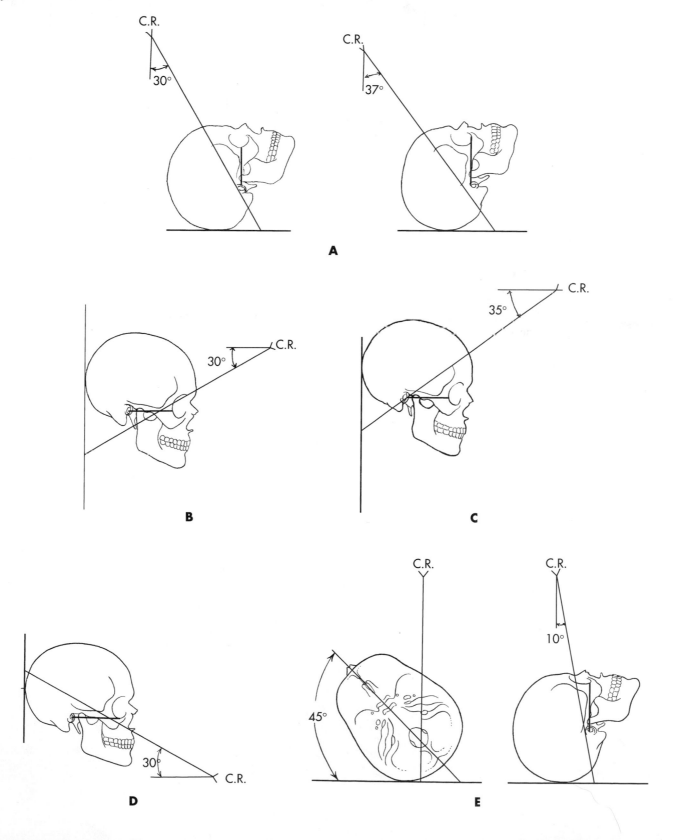

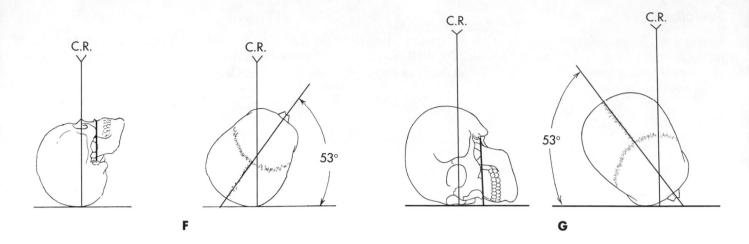

F

G

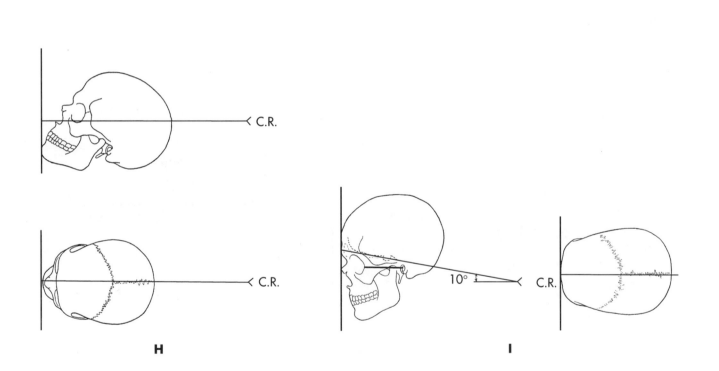

H

I

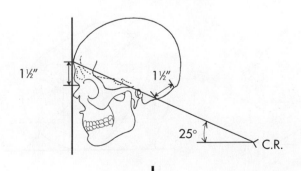

J

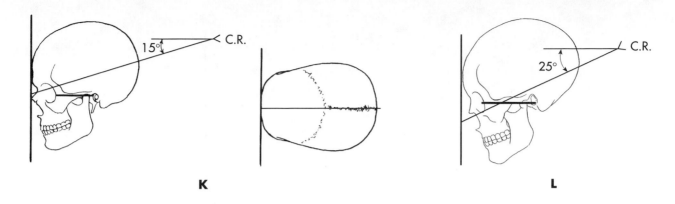

K

L

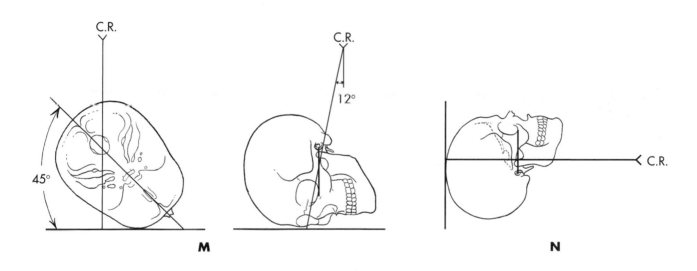

M

N

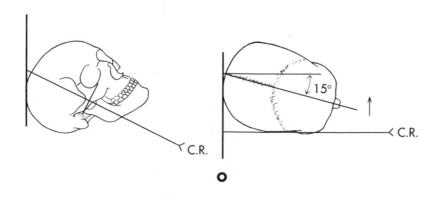

O

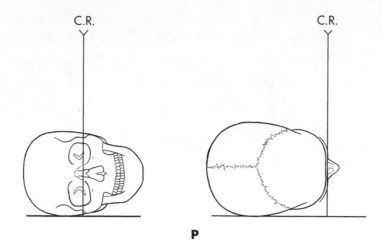

P

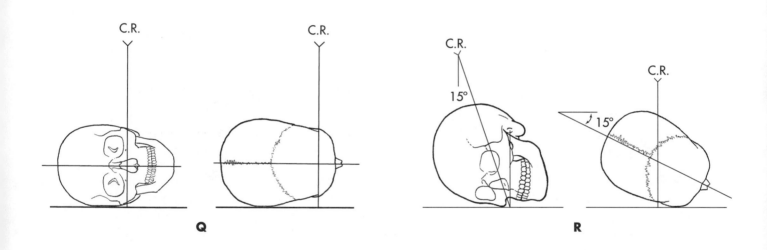

Q

R

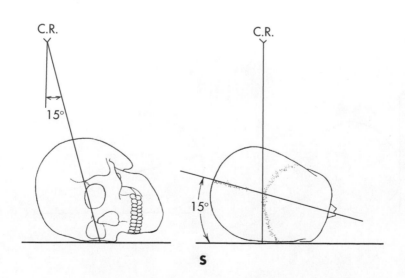

S

_____ 1. Parietoacanthial projection (Waters method)

_____ 2. Full basal projection of the cranium

_____ 3. AP axial projection (cranium, Towne method)

_____ 4. AP axial projection demonstrating facial bones

_____ 5. PA axial projection (cranium, Haas method)

_____ 6. PA axial projection (cranium, Caldwell method)

_____ 7. PA projection to demonstrate sphenoidal sinuses

_____ 8. Orbitoparietal oblique projection (Rhese method)

_____ 9. Parieto-orbital oblique projection (Rhese method)

_____ 10. Demonstrates one temporomandibular joint (TMJ)

_____ 11. Best projection for demonstrating the maxillary sinuses

_____ 12. Tangential projection for demonstrating an individual zygomatic arch

_____ 13. Petrous ridges should be projected immediately below the maxillae

_____ 14. Demonstrates the mastoid air cells of the side closest to the cassette

_____ 15. Lateral projection and central ray alignment for demonstrating the nasal bones

_____ 16. Lateral projection and central ray alignment for demonstrating the facial bones

_____ 17. Orbitomeatal line (OML) should form an angle of 37 degrees with the cassette

_____ 18. Petrous ridges should be projected into the lower one third of the orbits

_____ 19. Shows a profile image of the part of the petromastoid closest to the cassette

_____ 20. Axiolateral oblique projection (petromastoid portion, Arcelin method [anterior profile])

_____ 21. Axiolateral oblique projection (petromastoid portion, Stenvers method [posterior profile])

_____ 22. AP axial projection and central ray alignment for demonstrating bilateral zygomatic arches

_____ 23. AP axial projection and central ray alignment for demonstrating TMJs

_____ 24. Produces a slightly oblique tangential image of one zygomatic arch free from superimposed shadows

_____ 25. Central ray should enter 2 inches (5 cm) posterior to and 2 inches (5 cm) superior to the upside EAM

Answers to Exercises

CHAPTER 14 Mouth and Salivary Glands

Review

1. A. Posterior arch
   B. Anterior arch
   C. Tonsil
   D. Hard palate
   E. Uvula
   F. Soft palate
   G. Tongue
2. A. Orifice of the submandibular duct
   B. Tongue
   C. Frenulum of the tongue
   D. Sublingual fold
3. A. Parotid duct
   B. Sublingual ducts
   C. Submandibular duct
   D. Sublingual gland
   E. Parotid gland
   F. Submandibular gland
4. A. Muscle tissue
   B. Ramus of mandible
   C. Parotid gland
   D. Tongue
   E. Dens
   F. Atlas
   G. Spinal cord
5. A. Mandible
   B. Oropharynx
   C. Cervical vertebral body
   D. Sublingual gland
   E. Submandibular gland
   F. Tip of parotid gland
6. Mouth
7. The process of chewing and grinding food into small pieces
8. Teeth
9. To soften food, keep the mouth moist, and contribute digestive enzymes
10. Parotid, sublingual, and submandibular
11. Radiographic examination of the salivary glands and ducts with the use of a contrast medium
12. Water-soluble, iodinated medium
13. Salivary gland pairs are in close proximity.
14. To detect any condition demonstrable without the use of a contrast medium and to establish the optimal exposure factors
15. Tangential, lateral, and axial (intraoral method) projections
16. c
17. c
18. c
19. b
20. True
21. True
22. False (Only one parotid gland can be demonstrated with each tangential projection.)
23. a. Tangential projection
    b. Parotid
    c. The patient can fill the mouth with air and then puff the cheeks out as much as possible.
24. a. Lateral projection
    b. Parotid
    c. Parotid
25. a. Lateral projection
    b. Submandibular
    c. Submandibular

Self-Test: Mouth and Salivary Glands

1. a	5. b	9. c	13. a
2. a	6. d	10. d	14. c
3. b	7. b	11. a	15. b
4. a	8. a	12. a	

CHAPTER 15 Anterior Part of the Neck

Review

1. A. Nasal septum
   B. Nasopharynx
   C. Uvula
   D. Epiglottis
   E. Vocal folds
   F. Larynx
   G. Laryngeal pharynx
   H. Soft palate
   I. Piriform recess
   J. Rima glottidis
2. A. Soft palate
   B. Nasopharynx
   C. Uvula
   D. Oropharynx
   E. Epiglottis
   F. Vocal cords
   G. Larynx
   H. Hard palate
   I. Hyoid bone
   J. Laryngeal pharynx
   K. Trachea
   L. Thyroid cartilage
   M. Esophagus

3. A. Superior parathyroid gland
   B. Thyroid gland
   C. Inferior parathyroid gland
   D. Esophagus
   E. Thyroid cartilage
   F. Isthmus of the thyroid
   G. Trachea
4. A. Hyoid bone
   B. Thyroid cartilage
   C. Trachea
5. A. Base of the tongue
   B. Epiglottis
   C. Vestibular fold (false vocal cord)
   D. Rima glottidis (open)
   E. Rima glottidis (closed)
   F. Vocal fold (true vocal cord)
6. Posterior; anterior
7. Trachea
8. Esophagus
9. Thyroid; parathyroid
10. Pharynx
11. Nasopharynx
12. Oropharynx
13. Larynx
14. Glottis
15. AP projection; lateral projection
16. Breathing, phonation, stress maneuvers, and swallowing
17. a. Supine
    b. Upright
18. Laryngeal prominence
19. a. Level of the external acoustic meatuses
    b. Level of the mandibular angles
    c. Level of the laryngeal prominence
20. A. Air-filled pharynx
    B. Hyoid bone
    C. Laryngeal structures
    D. Trachea

Self-Test: Anterior Part of the Neck

1. c	6. d
2. a	7. b
3. d	8. b
4. b	9. b
5. c	10. b

CHAPTER 16 Digestive System: Abdomen, Liver, Spleen, and Biliary Tract
SECTION 1 Anatomy of the Abdomen, Liver, Spleen, and Biliary Tract

Exercise 1

1. A. Left lobe of the liver
   B. Falciform ligament
   C. Right lobe of the liver
   D. Gallbladder
   E. Ascending colon
   F. Ileum
   G. Appendix
   H. Diaphragm
   I. Esophagus
   J. Stomach
   K. Spleen
   L. Pancreas
   M. Descending colon
   N. Transverse colon
   O. Small intestine
   P. Urinary bladder
2. A. Tongue
   B. Sublingual gland
   C. Submandibular gland
   D. Gallbladder
   E. Biliary ducts
   F. Visceral surface of the liver
   G. Veriform appendix
   H. Parotid gland
   I. Pharynx
   J. Esophagus
   K. Stomach
   L. Spleen
   M. Pancreas
   N. Large intestine
   O. Small intestine
3. A. Hepatopancreatic ampulla
   B. Cystic duct
   C. Right lobe of the liver
   D. Gallbladder
   E. Liver
   F. Falciform ligament
   G. Quadrate lobe of the liver
   H. Left lobe of the liver
   I. Left hepatic duct
   J. Caudate lobe of the liver
   K. Common hepatic duct
   L. Common bile duct
   M. Pancreatic duct
   N. Pancreas
   O. Duodenum
4. A. Cut surface of the liver
   B. Gallbladder
   C. Cystic duct
   D. Right kidney
   E. Common hepatic duct
   F. Common bile duct
   G. Spleen
   H. Left kidney
   I. Pancreas
   J. Duodenum
5. A. Liver
   B. Duodenum
   C. Stomach
   D. Inferior vena cava
   E. Right kidney
   F. Aorta
   G. Pancreas
   H. Left kidney
   I. Spleen

Exercise 2

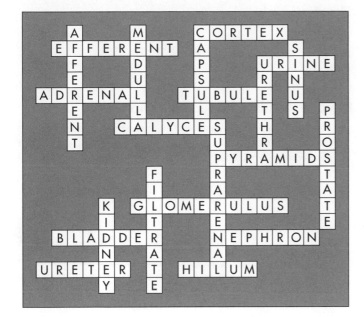

Exercise 3

1. l	6. g	11. o
2. p	7. j	12. e
3. a	8. f	13. m
4. d	9. h	14. c
5. k	10. n	15. i

Exercise 4

1. Urinary
2. Kidney
3. Suprarenal
4. Hilum
5. Medial
6. T12
7. Nephron
8. Cortex
9. Glomerular
10. Glomerulus
11. Renal
12. Afferent; efferent
13. Glomerular filtrate
14. Calyces
15. Calyces
16. Pelvis
17. Ureters
18. Urinary bladder
19. Urethra
20. Prostate

Exercise 5: Venipuncture and IV Contrast Media Administration

1. b
2. a
3. b
4. c
5. c

6. a
7. b
8. a.
9. b, d, g, h
10. Using tincture of iodine 1%–2% or isopropyl 70%, wipe the skin with a circular motion covering an area that is approximately 2 inches in diameter without lifting the swab from the skin until the process is completed.
11. 6 to 8 inches
12. Bevel-up
13. 45 degrees
14. The vein has been successfully penetrated by the needle.
15. Remove the needle and apply direct pressure to the puncture site.
16. c
17. c
18. b
19. a, b, c, d
20. a, b, c, e, f

SECTION 2 **Positioning of the Urinary System**

Exercise 1: Excretory Urography

1. Urography
2. d
3. a, b, c, e
4. a, c, e, f, j, k
5. a
6. a, c, e, g
7. To distend the stomach with gas, thus providing a negative background density that better demonstrates renal structures
8. Inappropriate abdominal pressure might retard the excretion of fluid from the kidneys and might cause distortion of ureteral structures.
9. To retard the flow of opacified urine into the bladder, allowing renal structures to be better filled and demonstrated
10. The anterior surface of the lower abdomen, about 2 inches (5 cm) above the pubic symphysis
11. Rapid releasing of the ureteral compression device might rupture some of the viscera within the pelvis.
12. Increased doses of contrast agents and the use of contrast media of higher concentrations produce better demonstration of ureters.
13. To demonstrate the mobility of the kidneys
14. Patient data, side marker, time-interval, and position indicator
15. Elastic waistbands in the underwear can produce unwanted densities in the image because of soft-tissue skin folds.
16. c
17. b, c, d, e, h
18. d
19. a
20. b
21. c
22. b
23. True
24. True
25. False (Postinjection radiographs are most often obtained with the patient supine.)
26. d
27. c
28. a

29. c
30. c
31. b
32. A. Renal calyces
    B. Renal pelvis
    C. Abdominal ureter
    D. Pelvic ureter
    E. Urinary bladder
33. b
34. a
35. c
36. c
37. b
38. a
39. Midcoronal
40. Arms extended in front of the patient, elbows flexed, and hands placed under the head
41. Pelvis and lumbar vertebrae
42. Expiration
43. Short
44. Supine
45. Midcoronal
46. a
47. b
48. True
49. False (The exposure should be made at the end of expiration.)
50. True

Exercise 2: Retrograde Urography

1. False (Contrast agents are injected into a selected renal pelvis by means of catheters that pass through the urethra, the bladder, and the ureter to the selected kidney.)
2. False (Special cystoscopic–radiographic tables are used for retrograde studies.)
3. c
4. c
5. a
6. The urologist intravenously injects a color dye, and the function of each kidney is determined by the time required for the dye substance to appear in the urine as it passes through the respective catheter.
7. A preliminary radiograph showing catheter insertion, a pyelogram, and a ureterogram
8. By retarding the excretion of the contrast medium from the kidney, the filling of the renal pelvis is enhanced.
9. b
10. a

Exercise 3: Retrograde Cystography

1. By means of a catheter passed through the urethra into the bladder
2. d
3. b
4. c
5. b
6. c
7. b
8. a
9. b
10. b
11. c
12. b

13. c
14. c
15. a, b
16. a
17. b
18. d
19. b
20. c

Exercise 4: Male Cystourethrography

1. The radiographic examination of the urinary bladder and urethra after the introduction of a contrast medium by means of a catheter inserted into the bladder
2. A catheter is inserted through the urethral canal into the bladder.
3. d
4. c
5. d
6. True
7. True
8. True
9. False (Only the bladder and urethra need to be demonstrated in their entirety.)
10. A. Bladder
    B. Prostatic urethra
    C. Membranous urethra
    D. Spongy (cavernous) urethra

Exercise 5: Identifying Urinary System Radiographs

1. d   6. b
2. a   7. a
3. b   8. a
4. b   9. b
5. a   10. d

Self-Test: Anatomy and Positioning of the Urinary System

1. a   10. d   18. c
2. b   11. a   19. d
3. c   12. b   20. a
4. b   13. a   21. c
5. d   14. b   22. a
6. c   15. d   23. c
7. c   16. b   24. d
8. b   17. b   25. d
9. c

CHAPTER 19 Reproductive System
SECTION 1 Anatomy of the Reproductive System

Exercise 1

1. A. Fundus
   B. Round ligament
   C. Ovarian ligament
   D. Uterine tube
   E. Ovary

2. A. Uterine tube (cut)
    B. Cervix
    C. Uterine ostium
    D. Rectum
    E. Ovary
    F. Uterine tube
    G. Uterus
    H. Round ligament (cut)
    I. Urinary bladder
    J. Pubic symphysis
    K. Urethral orifice
    L. Vaginal orifice
3. Ovaries
4. Ova
5. Uterine (or fallopian)
6. Two
7. Uterus
8. Fundus, body, isthmus, and cervix
9. Cervix
10. 1. e
    2. a
    3. b
    4. d
    5. c

Exercise 2

1. A. Testicular artery
    B. Ductus deferens
    C. Epididymis
    D. Head of the epididymis
    E. Testis
2. A. Sacrum
    B. Rectum
    C. Prostate
    D. Testes
    E. Bladder
    F. Pubis
    G. Urethra
3. A. Ureter
    B. Ductus deferens
    C. Bladder
    D. Seminal vesicle
    E. Ampulla
    F. Prostate
    G. Epididymis
    H. Testis
4. Testes (or testicles)
5. Spermatozoa
6. Epididymis
7. Ductus deferens
8. Ejaculatory
9. Prostate
10. Urethra

SECTION 2 Radiography of the Reproductive System

Exercise 1: Radiography of the Female Reproductive System

1. 1. a
    2. a
    3. b
    4. a
    5. b
    6. b
2. 1. b
    2. b
    3. d
    4. e
    5. c, e, f
    6. c, f
    7. f
    8. a, b, d, e
    9. a, b
    10. c
    11. f
    12. e
    13. c, e, f
    14. f
    15. c
3. i. d
    ii. c
    iii. b
    iv. b
    v. a

Exercise 2: Radiography of the Male Reproductive System

1. Water-soluble, iodinated
2. To improve radiographic contrast of examined structures
3. Prostate
4. Prone (because it places the prostate closer to the cassette and the sacrococcygeal vertebrae farther from the cassette)
5. 20 to 25 degrees cephalad

Self-Test: Reproductive System

1. a	6. c	11. d
2. c	7. c	12. b
3. b	8. a	13. b
4. a	9. d	14. c
5. b	10. d	15. b

CHAPTER 20 **Skull**
SECTION 1 **Osteology of the Skull**

Exercise 1

1. A. Parietal bone
   B. Glabella
   C. Greater wing of the sphenoid
   D. Nasal bone
   E. Temporal bone
   F. Zygomatic bone
   G. Perpendicular plate of the ethmoid
   H. Vomer
   I. Maxilla
   J. Frontal bone
   K. Sphenoid bone
   L. Lacrimal bone
   M. Ethmoid bone
   N. Middle nasal concha
   O. Infraorbital foramen
   P. Inferior nasal concha
   Q. Anterior nasal spine
   R. Mandible
2. A. Frontal bone
   B. Sphenoid bone
   C. Glabella
   D. Nasal bone
   E. Lacrimal bone
   F. Ethmoid bone
   G. Anterior nasal spine (acanthion)
   H. Zygomatic bone (zygoma)
   I. Temporal process
   J. Maxilla
   K. Mental foramen
   L. Mandible
   M. Bregma
   N. Coronal suture
   O. Parietal bone
   P. Squamosal suture
   Q. Lambda
   R. Lambdoidal suture
   S. Occipital bone
   T. External occipital protuberance (inion)
   U. Mastoid process
   V. Temporal bone
   W. External acoustic meatus
   X. Styloid process
3. A. Orbital plate
   B. Lesser wing
   C. Greater wing
   D. Optic groove
   E. Foramen ovale
   F. Foramen spinosum
   G. Temporal bone
   H. Petrous portion
   I. Clivus
   J. Occipital bone
   K. Crista galli
   L. Cribriform plate
   M. Optic canal and foramen
   N. Tuberculum sellae

O. Anterior clinoid process
P. Sella turcica
Q. Posterior clinoid process
R. Foramen lacerum
S. Dorsum sellae
T. Jugular foramen
U. Hypoglossal canal
V. Foramen magnum

4. A. Frontal bone
   B. Frontal sinus
   C. Crista galli
   D. Nasal bone
   E. Ethmoid bone
   F. Vomer
   G. Maxilla
   H. Parietal bone
   I. Sphenoidal sinus
   J. Petrous portion
   K. Internal acoustic meatus
   L. Occipital bone
   M. Squamous portion of the temporal bone
   N. Clivus
   O. Pterygoid hamulus
   P. Palatine bone
5. A. Frontal squama
   B. Supraorbital foramen
   C. Supraorbital margin
   D. Glabella
   E. Nasal spine
   F. Superciliary arch
   G. Frontal eminence
6. A. Superior nasal concha
   B. Middle nasal concha
   C. Perpendicular plate
   D. Crista galli
   E. Ethmoidal sinus
   F. Air cells in the labyrinth
   G. Cribriform plate
7. A. Parietal
   B. Frontal
   C. Frontal
   D. Sphenoid
   E. Occipital
   F. Occipital
   G. Mastoid
   H. Temporal
8. A. Anterior clinoid processes
   B. Posterior clinoid processes
   C. Dorsum sellae
   D. Lateral pterygoid lamina
   E. Pterygoid hamulus
   F. Optic canal and foramen
   G. Lesser wing
   H. Superior orbital fissure
   I. Greater wing
9. A. Squama
   B. Foramen magnum
   C. Basilar portion
   D. Occipital condyle
   E. External occipital protuberance (inion)

10. A. Squamous portion
    B. Mastoid portion
    C. External acoustic meatus
    D. Tympanic portion
    E. Styloid process
    F. Mandibular fossa
    G. Articular tubercle
    H. Zygomatic process
    I. Petrous portion
11. A. External acoustic meatus
    B. Cartilage
    C. Tympanic membrane
    D. Auditory ossicles
    E. Semicircular canals
    F. Stapes (in oval window)
    G. Internal acoustic meatus
    H. Cochlear nerve
    I. Cochlea
    J. Round window
    K. Auditory (Eustachian) tube
    L. Nasopharynx
    M. External acoustic meatus
    N. Auditory tube
12. A. Neck
    B. Condyle
    C. Alveolar process
    D. Mental foramen
    E. Symphysis
    F. Coronoid process
    G. Ramus
    H. Body
    I. Mental protuberance
    J. Angle
    K. Gonion
13. A. Body
    B. Greater cornu
    C. Lesser cornu

Exercise 2

Exercise 3

1. a	6. f	11. e	16. a
2. a	7. b	12. f	17. b
3. c	8. d	13. e	18. d
4. d	9. f	14. d	19. d
5. d	10. b	15. e	20. d

Exercise 4

1. m	6. n	11. g
2. q	7. r	12. j
3. i	8. l	13. f
4. c	9. k	14. b
5. e	10. p	15. s

Exercise 5

1. i	6. o	11. a
2. g	7. f	12. j
3. e	8. b	13. l
4. d	9. n	14. k
5. c	10. m	15. p

Exercise 6

1. Cranial; facial
2. Frontal (1); ethmoid (1); parietal (2); sphenoid (1); temporal (2); and occipital (1)
3. Nasal (2); lacrimal (2); maxillae (2); zygomatic (2); palatine (2); inferior nasal conchae (2); vomer (1); and mandible (1)
4. Mesocephalic (47 degrees); brachycephalic (54 degrees); and dolichocephalic (40 degrees)
5. Flat
6. Diploe
7. Bregma; lambda
8. Bregma
9. Lambda
10. Frontal
11. Ethmoid
12. Parietal
13. Eminence
14. Sagittal
15. Coronal
16. Occipital
17. Lambdoidal
18. Sphenoid
19. Occipital
20. Basilar
21. Foramen magnum
22. Sphenoid
23. C1 vertebra (atlas)
24. Sphenoid
25. Temporal
26. Tympanic
27. Mastoid
28. Petrous portion (pars petrosa, petrous pyramid)
29. Temporal
30. Auricle
31. Malleus (hammer); incus (anvil); stapes (stirrup)
32. Temporal
33. Temporal
34. Nasal
35. Lacrimal

36. Maxilla
37. Maxillary sinus
38. Alveolar process
39. Maxillae
40. Acanthion
41. Zygomatic
42. Zygomatic
43. Palatine
44. Inferior nasal conchae
45. Vomer
46. Mandible
47. Ramus
48. Hyoid
49. Condyle; coronoid
50. Condyle

SECTION 2 **Radiography of the Skull**

Exercise 1: Skull Topography

1. A. Angle of the mandible (gonion)
   B. Infraorbitomeatal margin
   C. Outer canthus
   D. Midsagittal plane
   E. Glabella
   F. Interpupillary line
   G. Inner canthus
   H. Nasion
   I. Acanthion
   J. Mental point
2. A. External acoustic meatus
   B. Angle of the mandible (gonion)
   C. Glabellomeatal line
   D. Orbitomeatal line
   E. Infraorbitomeatal line
   F. Acanthiomeatal line
   G. Glabelloalveolar line
   H. Glabella
   I. Nasion
   J. Acanthion
   K. Mental point
3. 1. c
   2. f
   3. a
   4. e
   5. h
   6. d
   7. b
   8. i
   9. g
4. 1. e
   2. b
   3. h
   4. d
   5. i
   6. g
   7. f
5. a. 7
   b. 8

Exercise 2: Positioning for the Cranium

1. c
2. a. Parallel
   b. Perpendicular
3. c
4. d
5. 2 inches (5 cm) above the external acoustic meatus
6. Perpendicular to a point approximately 2 inches (5 cm) above the external acoustic meatus
7. a
8. False (The central ray should enter at a point 2 inches [5 cm] superior to the external acoustic meatus.)
9. True
10. b, c, d, e, f, g, h, j
11. a. A support should be placed under the thorax to raise the inferior aspect of the head and to place the midsagittal plane parallel with the cassette.
    b. A radiolucent sponge should be placed under the head to make the midsagittal plane parallel with the cassette.
12. A. Orbital roof
    B. Sella turcica
    C. Sphenoidal sinus
    D. Petrous portion of the temporal bone
    E. Temporomandibular joint
    F. External acoustic meatus
    G. Mandibular rami
13. a. Perpendicular
    b. Perpendicular
14. c
15. 1. a
    2. b
    3. d
    4. c
16. Nasion
17. Nasion
18. Stop breathing.
19. a, c, g, h, i
20. A. Dorsum sellae
    B. Superior orbital margin
    C. Sphenoid plane
    D. Petrous ridge
    E. Ethmoidal sinus
    F. Inferior orbital margin
    G. Crista galli
21. a. Perpendicular
    b. Perpendicular
22. Perpendicularly
23. Cephalically
24. a
25. c
26. a, c, g, h, j
27. a. 15 degrees cephalad (The petrous ridges lie in the lower one third of the orbits.)
    b. Perpendicularly (The petrous ridges fill the orbits.)
28. d
29. c
30. Orbitomeatal; infraorbitomeatal
31. a
32. d
33. c

34. b, f, g, i
35. A. Parietal bone
    B. Occipital bone
    C. Foramen magnum
    D. Petrous ridge
    E. Posterior clinoid process
    F. Dorsum sellae
36. True
37. False (Hypersthenic patients must be either prone or upright.)
38. c
39. a
40. b
41. c
42. a, c, g, i
43. A. Occipital bone
    B. Foramen magnum
    C. Petrous ridge
    D. Posterior clinoid process
    E. Dorsum sellae
44. a. Perpendicular
    b. Parallel
45. Infraorbitomeatal
46. On the midsagittal plane of the throat between the angles of the mandible, passing through a point ³/₄ inch (1.9 cm) anterior to the level of the external acoustic meatus
47. a
48. b, e
49. a, d, f, h, i
50. A. Maxillary sinus
    B. Ethmoidal air cells
    C. Mandible
    D. Sphenoidal sinus
    E. Foramen spinosum
    F. Mandibular condyle
    G. Dens (odontoid process)
    H. Petrosa
    I. Mastoid process
51. c
52. a
53. b
54. b, e, h
55. A. Frontal bone and mandible
    B. Maxillary sinus
    C. Ethmoidal air cells
    D. Vomer
    E. Sphenoidal sinus
    F. Pharynx
    G. Foramen spinosum
    H. Mandibular condyle
    I. Mastoid air cells

Exercise 3: Positioning for the Sella Turcica

1. a. Parallel
   b. Perpendicular
   c. Parallel
2. At a point ³/₄ inch (1.9 cm) anterior to and 3/4 inch (1.9 cm) superior to the external acoustic meatus
3. Stop breathing.
4. a, b, c, d

5. A. Anterior clinoid process
   B. Posterior clinoid process
   C. Dorsum sellae
   D. Sella turcica
   E. Sphenoidal sinus

Exercise 4: Positioning for the Optic Canal and Foramen

1. b
2. b
3. a
4. True
5. True
6. False (The central ray should be directed perpendicularly through the affected orbit closer to the cassette.)
7. True
8. False (Incorrect angulation of the acanthiomeatal line causes longitudinal deviation from the preferred location of the optic canal and foramen. Any lateral deviation from the preferred location for the optic canal and foramen is caused by incorrect rotation of the head.)
9. b, e, f, g
10. A. Superior orbital margin
    B. Lateral orbital margin
    C. Optic canal and foramen
    D. Medial orbital margin
    E. Lesser wing of the sphenoid
    F. Ethmoidal sinus
    G. Inferior orbital margin
11. True
12. True
13. False (The orbitoparietal oblique projection is the AP oblique projection for the orbit. The PA oblique projection for the orbit is the parietoorbital oblique projection.)
14. False (The orbitoparietal oblique projection results in more radiation exposure to the lens of the eye than the parietoorbital oblique projection.)
15. True
16. Acanthiomeatal line
17. Midsagittal
18. a
19. b
20. c, e, f, g

Exercise 5: Evaluating Radiographs of the Skull

1. a. Fig. 20-40 (Certain structures of the skull are superimposed with their opposite side [orbital roofs, mandibular rami, mastoid regions, external acoustic meatuses, and temporomandibular joints], and no rotation is visible.)
   b. Fig. 20-39 (Cranial structures [orbital roofs, temporomandibular joints, and external acoustic meatuses] are longitudinally separated.)
   c. Fig. 20-38 (Cranial structures [orbital roofs, temporomandibular joints, and external acoustic meatuses] are laterally separated.)
   d. Fig. 20-39

2. a. Caudally 15 degrees
   b. In the lower one third of the orbits
   c. The distance from the lateral border of the skull to the lateral border of the orbit is not equal on both sides.
   d. The head is rotated, moving the occipital bone closer to the left shoulder. The midsagittal plane is not perpendicular to the cassette.
3. a. Perpendicular to the nasion
   b. The petrous ridges should fill the orbits.
   c. Yes
   d. The distance from the lateral border of the skull to the lateral border of the orbit is not equal on both sides.
   e. The head is rotated, moving the occipital bone closer to the right shoulder. The midsagittal plane is not perpendicular to the cassette.
4. a. Acceptable
   b. Unacceptable
   c. The head is rotated, moving the occipital bone closer to the left shoulder. The midsagittal plane is not perpendicular to the cassette.
   d. Perpendicularly
5. The mandibular symphysis does not superimpose the anterior frontal bone.
6. a. Fig. 20-47 (The optic foramen is demonstrated in the inferior and lateral quadrant of the orbit.)
   b. Fig. 20-46 (The position of the optic foramen is posterior to the lateral orbital margin.)
   c. Fig. 20-48 (The position of the optic foramen is too much toward the medial aspect of the orbit.)
7. a. The position of the optic foramen is deviated laterally from the preferred location.
   b. The angle formed by the midsagittal plane and the cassette was less than the required 53 degrees.
   c. Rotate the head, moving the occipital bone away from the cassette until the midsagittal plane forms an angle of 53 degrees with the cassette.

Self-Test: Osteology and Radiography of the Skull

1. a	19. b	37. a	54. a
2. d	20. c	38. d	55. d
3. a	21. d	39. c	56. d
4. b	22. b	40. b	57. c
5. c	23. a	41. d	58. d
6. d	24. b	42. d	59. c
7. d	25. a	43. b	60. d
8. d	26. c	44. c	61. a
9. b	27. d	45. b	62. b
10. a	28. c	46. c	63. d
11. c	29. b	47. a	64. d
12. d	30. d	48. a	65. c
13. a	31. b	49. c	66. c
14. c	32. d	50. c	67. b
15. a	33. b	51. a	68. c
16. b	34. c	52. c	69. c
17. a	35. c	53. d	70. b
18. c	36. c		

CHAPTER 21 Facial Bones

Radiography of the Facial Bones

Exercise 1: Positioning for Facial Bones and Nasal Bones

1. Lengthwise
2. Midsagittal
3. b
4. d
5. d
6. Perpendicularly
7. Halfway between the outer canthus and the EAM
8. a, b, d, g
9. A. Frontal sinus
   B. Nasal bone
   C. Sella turcica
   D. Maxillary sinus
   E. External acoustic meatus
   F. Maxilla
   G. Mandible
10. a. 37-degree angulation
    b. Perpendicular
11. b
12. a
13. a. Too far below maxillae (the maxillae will appear foreshortened)
    b. Immediately below the maxillae
    c. Superimpose maxillary sinuses
14. d, e
15. A. Orbit
    B. Zygomatic arch
    C. Maxillary sinus
    D. Maxilla
    E. Mandibular angle
16. Supine
17. Parietoacanthial; Waters
18. b
19. c
20. a
21. a
22. c
23. d, e
24. A. Orbit
    B. Zygomatic bone
    C. Maxillary sinus
25. a. Perpendicular
    b. Parallel
26. Two
27. Nasion
28. Perpendicular to the bridge of the nose at a point 1/2 inch (1.2 cm) distal to the nasion
29. c, d
30. A. Frontonasal (nasofrontal)
    B. Nasal bone
    C. Anterior nasal spine of the maxilla

Exercise 2: Positioning for Zygomatic Arches

1. True
2. False (The zygomatic arches should be free from overlying structures.)
3. False (The posterior cranium need not be included in the image.)
4. False (The midsagittal plane should be perpendicular to the cassette.)
5. c
6. c
7. c
8. a
9. a, b, d
10. True
11. True
12. Infraorbitomeatal
13. Perpendicularly to the infraorbitomeatal line and centered to the zygomatic arch at a point approximately 1½ inches (4 cm) posterior to the outer canthus
14. b
15. a. Perpendicular
    b. Perpendicular
16. a. 30 degrees caudad
    b. 37 degrees caudad
17. Nasion
18. True
19. False (Close beam restriction to zygomatic arches and adjacent structures may exclude the vertex.)
20. A. Occipital bone
    B. Mandible
    C. Zygomatic arch

Exercise 3: Positioning for the Mandible

1. b
2. a
3. Perpendicular
4. Stop breathing for the exposure.
5. b
6. b
7. True
8. False (The central portion of the mandible is superimposed with the cervical vertebrae.)
9. a, c
10. A. Condyle
    B. Mastoid process
    C. Fracture of the mandibular ramus
    D. Body
11. b
12. c
13. a
14. c
15. d
16. a
17. a, c, d
18. Fig. 21-18
19. Fig. 21-16
20. Fig. 21-18
21. Fig. 21-17
22. Fig. 21-16
23. Fig. 21-17
24. Fig. 21-17

25. NA
26. Figs. 21-16, 21-17, and 21-18
27. NA
28. NA
29. Figs. 21-16, 21-17, and 21-18
30. Fig. 21-18
31. Fig. 21-16
32. True
33. False (The neck should be extended to place the mandibular body parallel with the transverse axis of the cassette.)
34. True
35. A. Coronoid process
    B. Ramus
    C. Body
    D. Hyoid bone
    E. Angle

Exercise 4: Positioning for the Temporomandibular Joints (TMJs)

1. True
2. False (The head should be positioned the same way as for an AP projection, with the midsagittal plane perpendicular to the plane of the cassette.)
3. Occlusion of the incisors places the mandible in a position of protrusion in which the condyles are carried out of the mandibular fossae.
4. Any trauma to the mandible where the mandible is suspected to be fractured; because of the danger of fracture displacement
5. c
6. c
7. c
8. c
9. a, c
10. a, d
11. c
12. c
13. c
14. 15 degrees caudad
15. The TMJ closer to the cassette
16. In the mandibular fossa
17. False (To exit through the EAM closest to the cassette, the caudally directed central ray should enter about 11/2 inches [4 cm] superior to the upside EAM.)
18. True
19. False (Close beam restriction should surround the affected TMJ.)
20. A. Mandibular fossa
    B. Articular tubercle
    C. Condyle

Exercise 5: Evaluating Radiographs of Facial Bones

1. The mandibular rami are not superimposed, and the orbital roofs are not superimposed.
2. a. Fig. 21-26
   b. Fig. 21-24
   c. Fig. 21-25
3. a. The zygomatic arches are not symmetric, and the left zygomatic arch is superimposed with cranial structures.
   b. The midsagittal plane was not perpendicular to the cassette because the patient's head was slightly tilted.

4. a. The base of the occipital partially superimposes the mandible, and the mandibular rami are not seen without superimposition from surrounding structures.
   b. Reposition the head, ensuring that the forehead is in contact with the vertical grid device or x-ray table surface, to image the mandible without cranial superimposition.
5. a. The opposite side of the mandible superimposes the mandibular body.
   b. Position the head so that the uppermost side of the mandible will be projected above the mandibular body closer to the cassette.

Self-Test: Radiography of the Facial Bones

1. a	6. d	11. b	16. d
2. a	7. a	12. c	17. d
3. d	8. d	13. d	18. a
4. a	9. a	14. b	19. d
5. d	10. b	15. b	20. b

CHAPTER 22 Paranasal Sinuses

Review

1. Frontal, sphenoidal, ethmoidal, and maxillary
2. A. Sphenoidal
   B. Maxillary
   C. Frontal
   D. Ethmoidal
3. a
4. b
5. d
6. d
7. c
8. c
9. To demonstrate the presence or absence of fluid and to differentiate between shadows caused by fluid and those caused by other pathologic conditions
10. Underpenetration produces shadows simulating pathologic conditions that do not exist.
11. a. Parallel
    b. Perpendicular
12. d
13. a
14. d
15. d
16. a, b, c, d, e, f
17. A. Frontal sinus
    B. Sella turcica
    C. Sphenoidal sinus
    D. Ethmoidal sinuses
    E. Maxillary sinus
    F. Superimposed mandibular rami
18. c
19. c
20. c
21. a
22. a
23. b
24. c, d, e, g, h, k, l, m

25. A. Frontal sinus
    B. Ethmoidal sinuses
    C. Petrous ridge
    D. Sphenoidal sinuses
    E. Maxillary sinus
26. Maxillary
27. Superimposed with the maxillary sinuses
28. Foreshortened
29. Orbitomeatal
30. Mentomeatal
31. Acanthion
32. Immediately below the maxillary sinuses
33. One on each side, just inferior to the medial aspect of the orbital floor and superior to the roof of the maxillary sinuses
34. False (Only the chin should touch the vertical grid device.)
35. True
36. c, e, g, j, k
37. A. Frontal sinus
    B. Ethmoidal sinuses
    C. Foramen rotundum
    D. Maxillary sinus
    E. Petrous pyramid
    F. Mastoid air cells
38. Acanthion
39. Chin
40. Orbitomeatal
41. Sphenoidal
42. c, e, g, h, j, k
43. False (The head should rest on its vertex.)
44. False (The infraorbitomeatal line should be as close to parallel with the cassette as possible.)
45. True
46. True
47. True
48. False (To demonstrate the paranasal sinuses, close restriction of the beam to the sinus area may exclude the occipital bone.)
49. Sphenoidal and ethmoidal
50. The mandibular symphysis should superimpose the anterior frontal bone.
51. Anterior to the petrous ridges
52. The infraorbitomeatal line was not parallel with the cassette because the neck was not extended far enough (assuming the central ray was correctly directed).
53. The infraorbitomeatal line was not parallel with the cassette because the neck was extended too far or the vertical cassette holder was tilted too far toward the patient (assuming the central ray was correctly directed).
54. d, e, f
55. A. Maxillary sinus
    B. Ethmoidal sinus
    C. Mandible
    D. Vomer
    E. Sphenoidal sinus
    F. Mandibular condyle
    G. Petrosa
56. True
57. True
58. False (Close beam restriction should be limited to the sinus area.)
59. False (Respiration should be suspended for the exposure.)
60. a

61. a. Perpendicular to the nasion
    b. 10 degrees cephalad to the glabella
    c. Perpendicular to a point midway between the infraorbital margins and acanthion
62. c
63. a
64. b
65. b, c, f

Self-Test: Radiography of the Paranasal Sinuses

1. d	6. a	11. d	16. c	21. b
2. a	7. b	12. c	17. d	22. c
3. d	8. a	13. d	18. c	23. d
4. d	9. a	14. d	19. a	24. c
5. b	10. b	15. b	20. a	25. b

CHAPTER 23 **Temporal Bone**

Review

1. From true lateral, with the affected mastoid centered to the cassette, rotate the head until the midsagittal plane forms a 15-degree angle with the cassette.
2. a
3. c
4. d
5. 15 degrees caudad
6. Approximately 2 inches (5 cm) posterior and 2 inches (5 cm) above the uppermost external acoustic meatus
7. False (The head should be rotated 15 degrees from true lateral, moving the face closer to the cassette.)
8. False (The head should be rotated 15 degrees from true lateral, moving the face closer to the cassette.)
9. True
10. a, b, f, g, i, j
11. A. Internal and external acoustic meatus
    B. Mastoid air cells
    C. Mastoid process
    D. Mandibular condyle
12. Forehead, nose, and cheek
13. 12 degrees cephalad
14. d
15. d
16. d
17. c
18. A. Internal acoustic canal
    B. Arcuate eminence
    C. Mastoid air cells
    D. External acoustic meatus and canal
    E. Mandibular condyle
    F. Mastoid process
19. True
20. False (The midsagittal plane should form an angle of 45 degrees with the cassette.)
21. True
22. 10 degrees caudad
23. On the zygomatic bone approximately 1 inch (2.5 cm) anterior to and $^3/_4$ inch (1.9 cm) above the external acoustic meatus

24. d
25. b, e, f, g, h, j

Self-Test: Radiography of the Temporal Bone

1. d	6. c	11. b
2. d	7. a	12. c
3. d	8. d	13. b
4. d	9. d	14. b
5. c	10. a	15. a

CHAPTER 24 **Mammography**
SECTION 1 **Anatomy and Physiology of the Breast**

Exercise 1

1. A. Axillary prolongation (tail) of the breast
   B. Serratus anterior
   C. Pectoralis minor
   D. Pectoralis major (cut)
2. A. Fat
   B. Nipple
   C. Lactiferous tubules
   D. Fat
   E. Inframammary crease
   F. Pectoralis major
   G. Retromammary fat

Exercise 2

1. Mammary
2. Milk
3. Tail
4. Base
5. Nipple
6. Areola
7. 15; 20
8. Acini
9. Smaller
10. Involution
11. Fat
12. Lactiferous
13. Cooper's
14. Axilla
15. Sternum

Exercise 3

1. h
2. g
3. b
4. e
5. i
6. f
7. d
8. c

SECTION 2 **Radiography of the Breast**

Exercise 1

1. Because the mammogram will record the slightest wrinkle in any cloth covering
2. These substances will resemble calcifications on the resultant image.
3. Craniocaudal and mediolateral oblique projections
4. To locate a nipple that is not in profile
5. Compress the breast with an approved mammographic compression device.
6. Place a radiopaque marker such as a BB on the breast overlying the mass.
7. To evaluate whether or not sufficient breast tissue is demonstrated
8. Nipple and chest wall, or edge of the image, whichever comes first
9. 1 cm
10. Clean the image receptor surface and face guard with a disinfectant.

Exercise 2

1. a
2. d
3. c
4. b

Exercise 3

1. b
2. a, b, c, d
3. b, d
4. a, b, c
5. d
6. a, b, c, d
7. a
8. b
9. c
10. a

Exercise 4

1. a
2. a
3. b
4. c
5. b
6. a
7. d
8. d

Self-Test: Mammography

1. a	6. d	11. b
2. c	7. a	12. a
3. d	8. c	13. c
4. d	9. c	14. c
5. b	10. c	15. a

CHAPTER 25 **Central Nervous System**
SECTION 1 **Anatomy of the Central Nervous System**

1. A. Cerebrum
   B. Corpus callosum
   C. Cerebrum
   D. Cerebellum
   E. Pituitary gland
   F. Medulla oblongata
   G. Cerebellum
   H. Pons
2. A. Gray substance
   B. White substance
   C. Posterior nerve root
   D. Anterior nerve root
3. A. Pons
   B. Medulla oblongata
   C. Spinal cord
   D. Dural sac for the cauda equina
4. A. Fourth ventricle
   B. Inferior horn
   C. Interventricular foramen
   D. Anterior horn
   E. Body of the lateral ventricle
   F. Third ventricle
   G. Posterior horn
   H. Cerebral aqueduct
5. A. Body of the lateral ventricle
   B. Anterior horn
   C. Inferior horn
6. A. Fourth ventricle
   B. Body of the lateral ventricle
   C. Third ventricle
   D. Anterior horn
   E. Inferior horn
   F. Lateral recess
   G. Posterior horn
7. Brain and spinal cord
8. Cerebrum, cerebellum, and brain stem
9. Diencephalon, midbrain (mesencephalon), pons, and medulla oblongata
10. Cerebellum, pons, and medulla oblongata
11. Cerebrum (forebrain)
12. Forebrain
13. Midbrain (mesencephalon)
14. Longitudinal fissure
15. Pituitary gland
16. Cerebellum
17. Medulla oblongata
18. Meninges
19. Pia mater
20. Dura mater
21. Lateral
22. Cerebrum (forebrain)
23. Interventricular
24. Monro
25. Cerebral aqueduct and aqueduct of Sylvius

SECTION 2 **Radiography of the Central Nervous System**

1. Radiographic examination of the spinal cord after the injection of a contrast medium into the subarachnoid space
2. L2-L3, L3-L4, and cisterna cerebellomedullaris (cisterna magna)
3. Extrinsic spinal cord compression
4. Nonionic, water-soluble (They provide good visualization of nerve roots and good enhancement for follow-up computerized tomography, and they are readily absorbed by the body.)
5. To prevent it from accidentally contacting the spinal needle
6. Explain details of the examination to the patient before beginning the procedure.
7. Prone and lateral recumbent with the spine flexed
8. Varying the angulation of the table
9. To compress the cisterna cerebellomedullaris, preventing the contrast medium from entering cranial structures
10. Cross-table lateral of the cervical spine

Self-Test: Central Nervous System

1. b	6. a	11. b
2. b	7. c	12. a
3. c	8. d	13. b
4. b	9. c	14. d
5. b	10. d	15. c

CHAPTER 26 **Circulatory System**
SECTION 1 **Anatomy of the Circulatory System**

Exercise 1

1. A. Superior sagittal sinus
   B. Transverse sinus
   C. Internal jugular vein
   D. Right subclavian artery and vein
   E. Superior vena cava
   F. Brachial artery and basilic vein
   G. Celiac axis (artery)
   H. Portal vein
   I. Renal artery and vein
   J. Superior mesenteric artery and vein
   K. Common iliac artery and vein
   L. Common femoral artery and vein
   M. Popliteal artery
   N. Anterior tibial artery
   O. Posterior tibial artery
   P. Anterior facial artery and vein
   Q. Common carotid artery
   R. Aortic arch
   S. Pulmonary artery and vein
   T. Aorta
   U. Inferior vena cava
   V. Inferior mesenteric vein
   W. Radial artery and cephalic vein
   X. Ulnar artery and basilic vein
   Y. Deep femoral artery
   Z. Superficial femoral artery
   AA. Popliteal vein
   BB. Large saphenous vein

2. A. Aortic arch
   B. Superior vena cava
   C. Right pulmonary artery
   D. Right pulmonary veins
   E. Right atrium
   F. Right atrioventricular (tricuspid) valve
   G. Right ventricle
   H. Inferior vena cava
   I. Descending aorta
   J. Left ventricle
   K. Left atrioventricular (bicuspid or mitral) valve
   L. Left lung
   M. Left atrium
3. A. Right coronary artery
   B. Left coronary artery
4. A. Coronary sinus
   B. Great cardiac vein
5. A. Capillaries
   B. Lungs
   C. Right atrium
   D. Right ventricle
   E. Liver
   F. Intestine
   G. Aorta
   H. Left atrium
   I. Left ventricle
   J. Stomach
   K. Spleen
   L. Pancreas
6. A. External carotid artery
   B. Internal carotid artery
   C. Right common carotid artery
   D. Right vertebral artery
   E. Right subclavian artery
   F. Brachiocephalic artery
   G. Brachial artery
   H. Radial artery
   I. Ulnar artery
   J. Left subclavian artery
   K. Left vertebral artery
   L. Left common carotid artery
   M. Thyroid
7. A. Axillary nodes
   B. Common iliac nodes
   C. Deep inguinal nodes
   D. Cervical nodes
   E. Thoracic duct
   F. Lumbar nodes
   G. Superior inguinal nodes

Exercise 2

1. Blood–vascular; lymphatic
2. Pulmonary; systemic
3. Pulmonary
4. Arteries
5. Veins
6. Arterioles
7. Capillaries
8. Venules
9. Venules
10. Pulmonary

11. Superior vena cava
12. Inferior vena cava
13. Myocardium
14. Endocardium
15. Epicardium
16. Left ventricle
17. Pericardial cavity
18. Atria
19. Ventricles
20. Atria
21. Ventricles
22. Tricuspid
23. Mitral; bicuspid
24. Right
25. Left
26. Left ventricle
27. Coronary
28. Cardiac
29. Right
30. Aorta
31. Iliac
32. Femoral
33. Popliteal
34. Tibial
35. Portal
36. Hepatic
37. Inferior vena cava
38. Pulmonary
39. Pulmonary
40. Pulmonary
41. Systole
42. Diastole
43. Common carotid; vertebral
44. Left common carotid
45. Subclavian
46. Basilar
47. Internal; external
48. Cerebral
49. Posterior cerebral
50. Jugular
51. Brachiocephalic
52. Subclavian
53. Brachial
54. Radial; ulnar
55. Forearm
56. Aorta (abdominal)
57. Brain
58. Heart
59. Thoracic
60. Subclavian; jugular

SECTION 2 **Radiography of the Circulatory System**

1. The risk of extravasation is reduced; most body parts can be reached for selective injection; the patient can be positioned as needed; and the catheter can be safely left in the body while the radiographs are being examined.
2. Seldinger
3. Femoral

4. b
5. b, c, g
6. b, d, e
7. The patient's legs should be elevated, and intravenous fluids may be administered.
8. To reduce the possibility of the aspiration of vomitus
9. To saturate the kidneys and minimize kidney damage from iodinated contrast media
10. T6
11. A. Brachiocephalic artery
    B. Ascending aorta
    C. Right coronary artery
    D. Intercostal arteries
    E. Left common carotid artery
    F. Left subclavian artery
    G. Left coronary artery
    H. Descending thoracic aorta
12. From the diaphragm to the aortic bifurcation
13. Lateral
14. A. Hepatic artery
    B. Right renal artery
    C. Right common iliac artery
    D. Splenic artery
    E. Left renal artery
    F. Abdominal aorta
15. A. Celiac axis
    B. Superior mesenteric artery
    C. Abdominal aorta
16. AP
17. Expiration
18. A. Left gastric artery
    B. Hepatic artery
    C. Gastroduodenal artery
    D. Splenic artery
    E. Celiac axis
19. To ensure exact positioning of the tube-part-film alignment and close collimation of the x-ray tube
20. Splenic
21. Proximally
22. Upper
23. a
24. b
25. b
26. A. Ulnar artery
    B. Posterior interosseous artery
    C. Brachial artery
    D. Right subclavian artery
27. In the superficial vein at the wrist (when demonstrating the entire upper limb) or at the elbow (when demonstrating the upper arm)
28. A. Cephalic vein
    B. Basilic vein
    C. Subclavian vein
29. Extended and internally rotated 30 degrees
30. A. Common iliac artery
    B. External iliac artery
    C. Profunda femoris artery
    D. Femoral artery
    E. Popliteal artery
    F. Anterior tibial artery
    G. Peroneal artery
    H. Posterior tibial artery

31. c
32. c
33. a
34. c
35. a
36. a. Capillary
    b. Arterial
    c. Venous
37. Infraorbitomeatal
38. Away from the injected side
39. a
40. b

Self-Test: Anatomy and Radiography of the Circulatory System

1. c	6. b	11. c	16. d
2. d	7. a	12. b	17. b
3. c	8. a	13. c	18. a
4. a	9. a	14. c	19. b
5. d	10. b	15. c	20. d

CHAPTER 27 Sectional Anatomy for Radiographers

Review

1. A. Frontal bone
   B. Superior sagittal sinus
   C. Parietal bone
   D. White matter
   E. Falx cerebri (longitudinal fissure)
2. A. Genu of the corpus callosum
   B. Internal capsule
   C. Basal nuclei
   D. Third ventricle
   E. Occipital lobe
   F. Longitudinal fissure
   G. Anterior horn of the lateral ventricle
   H. Caudate nucleus
   I. Thalamus
   J. Posterior horn of the lateral ventricle
3. A. Longitudinal fissure
   B. Middle cerebral artery
   C. Basilar artery
   D. Pons
   E. Fourth ventricle
   F. Cerebellum
   G. Frontal lobe
   H. Frontal sinus
   I. Anterior cerebral artery
   J. Posterior cerebral artery
   K. Mastoid air cells
4. A. Sphenoidal sinus
   B. Internal carotid artery
   C. Pars petrosa
   D. Auricle of the ear
   E. Ethmoidal sinuses
   F. Ocular bulb
   G. Optic nerve
   H. Temporal lobe
   I. Basilar artery
   J. Pons
   K. Cerebellum
5. A. Mandibular symphysis
   B. Hyoid
   C. Submandibular gland
   D. Common carotid artery
   E. Sternocleidomastoid muscle
   F. Internal jugular vein
   G. Epiglottic cartilage
   H. Laryngeal pharynx
6. A. Common carotid artery
   B. Thyroid gland
   C. Thyroid cartilage
   D. Larynx
   E. Pharynx
   F. Internal jugular vein
   G. Trapezius muscle
   H. Body of the T6 vertebra
   I. Vertebral artery
7. A. Lateral ventricle
   B. Third ventricle
   C. Optic chiasm
   D. Pituitary gland
   E. Sphenoidal sinus
   F. Clivus
   G. Nasopharynx
   H. Maxilla
   I. Tongue
   J. Corpus callosum
   K. Great cerebral vein (of Galen)
   L. Corpora quadrigemina
   M. Cerebral aqueduct
   N. Straight sinus
   O. Cerebellum
   P. Fourth ventricle
   Q. Pons
   R. Basilar artery
   S. Cervical spinal cord
   T. C2 vertebra
8. A. Superior sagittal sinus
   B. Longitudinal fissure
   C. Corpus callosum
   D. Lateral ventricle
   E. Septum pellucidum
   F. Lateral fissure
   G. Sphenoidal sinus
   H. Mandibular ramus
   I. Masseter muscle
   J. Submandibular gland
   K. Caudate nucleus
   L. Basal nuclei
   M. Third ventricle
   N. Optic chiasm
   O. Pituitary gland
   P. Internal carotid artery
   Q. Nasopharynx
   R. Medial pterygoid muscle
   S. Oropharynx

9. A. Superior sagittal sinus
   B. Lateral ventricle
   C. Third ventricle
   D. External acoustic canal
   E. Parotid gland
   F. Dens
   G. Vertebral artery
   H. Internal carotid artery
   I. Thalamus
   J. Cranial nerves (in the internal acoustic canal)
   K. Sternocleidomastoid muscle
10. A. Lateral ventricle
    B. Pineal body
    C. Superior and inferior colliculi
    D. Auricle
    E. Middle cerebellar peduncle
    F. Medulla oblongata
    G. Cervical spinal cord
    H. Corpus callosum (splenium)
    I. Cerebral aqueduct
    J. Cerebellum
    K. Mastoid region
11. A. Manubrium
    B. Brachiocephalic artery
    C. Right brachiocephalic vein
    D. Trachea
    E. Esophagus
    F. Scapula
    G. Left common carotid artery
    H. Left brachiocephalic vein
    I. Left subclavian artery
    J. Left lung
12. A. Sternum
    B. Ascending aorta
    C. Superior vena cava
    D. Right pulmonary artery
    E. Right primary bronchus
    F. Azygos vein
    G. Body of the T5 vertebra
    H. Pulmonary trunk
    I. Left pulmonary artery
    J. Descending aorta
    K. Scapula
13. A. Serratus anterior muscle
    B. Liver
    C. Right atrium
    D. Right ventricle
    E. Sternum
    F. Left ventricle
    G. Esophagus
    H. Latissimus dorsi muscle
    I. Descending aorta
    J. Azygos vein
    K. Inferior vena cava

14. A. Pharynx
    B. Tongue
    C. Epiglottis
    D. Trachea
    E. Left brachiocephalic vein
    F. Manubrium
    G. C2 vertebra
    H. Spinal cord
    I. Intervertebral disk
    J. Brachiocephalic artery
    K. Aortic arch
    L. Right pulmonary artery
15. A. Spinal cord
    B. Sternocleidomastoid muscle
    C. Right lung
    D. Tracheal bifurcation
    E. Heart
    F. Left subclavian artery
    G. Clavicle
    H. Acromion
    I. Humeral head
    J. Aortic arch
    K. Pulmonary trunk
16. A. Liver
    B. Lower lobe of the right lung
    C. Stomach
    D. Diaphragm
    E. Spleen
    F. Esophagus
    G. Aorta
17. A. Caudate lobe
    B. Right lobe of the liver
    C. Portal vein
    D. Quadrate lobe
    E. Ligamentum teres
    F. Left lobe of the liver
    G. Stomach
    H. Aorta
    I. Spleen
    J. Crus of the diaphragm
    K. Inferior vena cava
18. A. Superior mesenteric artery
    B. Right lobe of the liver
    C. Inferior vena cava
    D. Right kidney
    E. Crus of the diaphragm
    F. Stomach
    G. Rectus abdominis muscle
    H. Body of the pancreas
    I. Left colic flexure
    J. Aorta
19. A. Inferior vena cava
    B. Right lobe of the liver
    C. Aorta
    D. Left kidney
    E. Stomach (with contrast)
    F. Tail of the pancreas
    G. Spleen

20. A. Psoas major muscle
    B. Iliacus (iliac) muscle
    C. Ureter
    D. Rectus abdominis muscle
    E. Anterior superior iliac spine (ASIS)
    F. Ilium
    G. Sacroiliac (SI) joint
21. A. Femoral vessels
    B. Pubic symphysis
    C. Bladder
    D. Acetabulum
    E. Head of the femur
    F. Rectum
    G. Gluteus
22. A. Obturator externus muscle
    B. Obturator internus muscle
    C. Greater trochanter
    D. Prostate
    E. Rectum
    F. Spermatic cord
    G. Corpora cavernosa (of the penis)
    H. Pubic bone
    I. Femoral vessels
    J. Femoral head
    K. Gluteus maximus muscle
    L. Ischium
23. A. Aorta
    B. Rectus abdominis muscle
    C. Bladder
    D. Pubic bone
    E. Corpora cavernosa
    F. Cauda equina
    G. L4 vertebra
    H. Sacrum
    I. Rectum
    J. Coccyx
    K. Prostatic urethra (within the prostate)
    L. Corpus spongiosum
    M. Testicles (testes)
24. A. Sigmoid colon
    B. Bladder
    C. Ductus deferens

D. Prostate
E. Gracilis muscle
F. Psoas muscle
G. Iliacus (iliac) muscle
H. Ilium
I. Gluteus medius muscle
J. Gluteus minimus muscle
K. Acetabulum
L. Pubic ramus
M. Corpus spongiosum
N. Scrotum

APPENDIX Supplemental Exercises for Skull Positioning
Skull Positioning Review

Exercise 1

1. o	6. m	11. b
2. n	7. a	12. e
3. p	8. f	13. a
4. n	9. m	14. a
5. c	10. f	15. f

Exercise 2

1. n	6. j	11. h
2. f	7. g	12. k
3. d	8. a	13. p
4. o	9. c	14. l
5. i	10. b	15. m

Exercise 3

1. H	8. F	14. S	20. E
2. N	9. G	15. P	21. M
3. A	10. R	16. Q	22. B
4. D	11. H	17. H	23. C
5. J	12. O	18. K	24. O
6. K	13. H	19. M	25. S
7. I			